# Personal Process in Child-Centred Play Therapy

*Personal Process in Child-Centred Play Therapy* provides a very specific exploration of the play therapy process from the personal perspective of the play therapist.

This volume examines the personal challenges, opportunities, losses and gains, and numerous obstacles that one has to negotiate through the course of both training to become a play therapist and working as a qualified clinician with children who have complex life difficulties. The book aims to offer a forum within which the role, function and process of the "personal" within play therapy can be explored. Bringing together a number of experienced play therapists, the book shares often deeply personal accounts of their experience of training and clinical practice. Chapters challenge the unspoken therapist taboos of shame, childhood trauma, vulnerability and grief, shining a light on the more hidden areas of therapist experience. Clinical issues around the unconscious process are also explored, but once again from the personal position of the play therapist, rather than the child.

With a unique and distinct perspective on the therapeutic process, this book is specifically intended for both trainee and experienced play therapists, but will be relevant to all psychotherapists involved in working therapeutically with children and young people.

**David Le Vay** is a qualified social worker and registered play therapist, dramatherapist and sandplay therapist. He has worked with children, who have experienced significant loss, trauma and abuse, as well as with their families and carers. He is also Senior Lecturer at Roehampton University and an approved BAPT play therapy supervisor.

**Elise Cuschieri** is Senior Lecturer and convenes the MA Play Therapy programme at the University of Roehampton. She is a BAPT-registered play therapist and works in the NHS and other sectors with children and their families who have experienced life-limiting illness, loss, trauma and abuse.

# Personal Process in Child-Centred Play Therapy

Edited by David Le Vay
and Elise Cuschieri

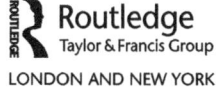
Routledge
Taylor & Francis Group

LONDON AND NEW YORK

Cover image: © Getty Images

First published 2023
by Routledge
4 Park Square, Milton Park, Abingdon, Oxon OX14 4RN

and by Routledge
605 Third Avenue, New York, NY 10158

Routledge is an imprint of the Taylor & Francis Group, an informa business

British Library Cataloguing-in-Publication Data

A catalogue record for this book is available from the British Library

Library of Congress Cataloging-in-Publication Data
A catalog record for this book has been requested

ISBN: 978-0-367-86160-5 (hbk)
ISBN: 978-0-367-86158-2 (pbk)
ISBN: 978-1-003-01727-1 (ebk)

DOI: 10.4324/9781003017271

Typeset in Times New Roman
by Apex CoVantage, LLC

In memory of Jan Vance, play therapist and contributor to our first text "Challenges in the Theory and Practice of Play Therapy", who died in March 2018.

# Contents

# Contributors

**Maria Victoria Aralde**

*Maria Victoria Aralde is a professionally qualified and accredited preschool teacher, filial therapist and play therapist. Her clinical practice is in a specialist bereavement service where she provides emotional support for children and families in their experiences related to life-limiting illness and/or bereavement.*

**Lisa Gordon Clark**

*Lisa is a BAPT-registered play therapist and clinical supervisor based in Wiltshire. Until 2020 she was Programme Convener for the Play Therapy MA at the University of Roehampton, where she still runs the 20-week Play Therapy Foundation Course. From 2017 to 2020, she was the External Examiner for the Play Therapy Master's programme at Queen Margaret University, Edinburgh. Lisa has been editor of the British Journal of Play Therapy since 2008.*

**Elise Cuschieri**

*Elise is Senior Lecturer and convenes the MA Play Therapy programme at the University of Roehampton. She is a BAPT-registered play therapist and works in the NHS with children and their families who have experienced life-limiting illness and loss. Elise has worked in other sectors with children and families who have been affected by trauma and abuse. Elise is also a BAPT-approved play therapy supervisor and has done training in filial therapy and child-parent relationship therapy.*

**Genene Grubb**

*Genene Grubb is a qualified play therapist who completed her MA Play Therapy at the University of Roehampton in 2019. Genene developed an interest in early intervention and therapeutic support after working with adolescents and adults across numerous psychiatric inpatient and community crisis settings. Currently, Genene works as a play therapist for two children's mental health charities.*

### Ann Marie John

*Ann Marie John is a dramatherapist, play therapist, systemic family psychothera-pist and supervisor. She currently works at the Tavistock and Portman Clinic, training family therapists, and as a clinician for Norfolk and Suffolk E.D. Ser-vice. She has a private practice specialising in ADHD, eating disorders and preventing parental alienation, and is an aspiring playwright.*

### Simon Kerr-Edwards

*Simon Kerr-Edwards is an independent play therapist, clinical supervisor and trainer and former dramatherapist who practices in Buckinghamshire, UK. He is a specialist in working with adopted children and their families and uses playful ways of exploring children's early life stories. His interest is in bringing creativity and improvisation into the clinical supervision relationship.*

### Lauren Shaw

*Lauren Shaw is a BAPT accredited play therapist with an MA in Play Therapy from the University of Roehampton. Delivering services to children, young people and families with complex needs, with a particular focus on adoption, domestic and sexual abuse, she employs a holistic approach to support and offers individual sessions, parental support and training.*

### Sue Topping

*Sue has worked with children and young people since the early 1990s in a career spanning playwork, youth work, sports coaching and strategic development in local government. Since 2011, Sue has worked in the charity sector as a trainer of adults and young people in the field of mental health and well-being, adding play therapy to her professional portfolio in 2018.*

### David Le Vay

*David is a qualified social worker and registered play therapist, dramatherapist and sandplay therapist. Since qualifying as a therapist in 1992, he has worked with children, who have experienced significant loss, trauma and abuse, as well as with their families and carers. He is also Senior Lecturer at Roehamp-ton University on their MA Play Therapy Programme and an approved BAPT play therapy supervisor.*

### Martine Wheeldon

*Martine Wheeldon is BAPT registered play therapist who qualified from the Uni-versity of Roehampton in 2018. Martine has experience working with clients in clinical, educational and most recently residential care settings. Martine is also trained in Developmental Dyadic Psychotherapy (DDP) and supports children, their parents and carers to build stronger attachments and explore early life experiences.*

## Francesca Wright

*Francesca Wright is a qualified and accredited play therapist with 3 years of experience of working with children, predominantly those who have experience of the care system. She also works within a refuge setting delivering play therapy and filial therapy programmes to children and their mothers who have fled domestic abuse.*

## Sarah Zehetmayr-McCall

*Sarah is a practising Christian, wife to Iain, and mother to Andrew, Maggie and Paddy. She qualified as Social Worker in 2001 and as a play therapist in 2018. Sarah currently works part-time for an adult hospice as a social worker and play therapist, as well as having a private practice in Wiltshire.*

# Preface

The idea for this book emerged out of a conversation between Elise and myself on a long-haul flight back to London from Ningbo, China, where we both had been presenting at a conference on "Playful Pedagogy", sharing ideas with an eclectic, international group of therapists, psychologists and sociologists about how to integrate creative, playful approaches into teaching within a higher education context. I recall the trip with great fondness; sitting drinking Longjing green tea with Elise by the serene waters of Moon Lake, an oasis of peace and calm within the otherwise rather frenetic life of the city. We just sat, immersed in a rather wonderful sense of cultural "otherness", and let the sounds, smells, tastes and sights wash over us like some kind of sensory shower. It was September 2018 and the world felt a very different place back then.

Perhaps it was the reflective spirit of Moon Lake, the creative stimulation of the conference, the travelling or simply the need to break up the relentless tedium of hours of airline food and in-flight entertainment, but our conversation turned to how we might be able to follow up our 2016 volume, *Challenges in the Theory and Practice of Play Therapy*, which explored some of the personal and professional challenges that play therapists are inevitably confronted with during the course of their clinical practice. Specifically, and perhaps as a sequential "next step" from our previous book, we were interested in the personal process of the therapist; an exploration of the therapeutic process from the personal perspective of the play therapist, both qualified and trainee. The therapeutic relationship, by definition, requires an exploration of the self and so we were interested in providing an insight into that process of personal exploration; the very personal challenges, opportunities, losses, gains and numerous obstacles that one has to negotiate through the course of both training to become a play therapist and of working as a qualified clinician with children with complex life difficulties. In many ways it felt a challenging concept for a therapy book, crossing boundaries around self-disclosure and giving voice to the unspoken, but then we would argue that to be working as "good enough" therapists we need to be cognisant and reflective as much upon our own process as we are upon that of the child's.

As a beginning point, Elise and I met in person with all our contributors, inviting everyone to bring with them an object that symbolised the subject matter of their chapter. It was a deeply moving, powerfully poignant process as we collectively became aware of the risks that we were all prepared to take with this project, sharing together very personal aspects of our lives and experiences and how these informed our work as play therapists. Important conversations were had about the process of self-disclosure and self-care, where our boundaries lay and what it would mean to put something in writing that could not be taken back. We soon realised that this would be a play therapy book like no other, and Elise and I felt privileged, honoured and humbled to be in the company of colleagues who felt brave enough to trust in us as editors and commit to the challenging process of this writing project.

Over the course of 2019, we met a couple more times as a group, exploring ways in which we could support each other through the process of writing. I had a six-month career break to go travelling, planned from the beginning of 2020, and my aim was to continue co-editing with Elise, from wherever in the world I happened to be. In October 2019, I was diagnosed with Parkinson's disease. In 2020 the world was hit by the global COVID-19 pandemic. In the summer of 2020, Elise took over convening the MA Play Therapy Programme, delivering an intense therapeutic training programme during the most challenging circumstances one could imagine. The irony of trying to write a book on personal process during this period was not lost on us. We were all, in various ways, impacted by the pandemic, grieving, furloughed, ill, struggling with home-teaching and home-working. Suddenly, we were all completely overwhelmed by personal process and to try and write about it, in the midst of such global and personal turmoil, seemed an almost paradoxically absurd endeavour.

But somehow, despite everything, we managed to just about keep the ship on course, and Elise and I would like to acknowledge and thank the tenacity, courage and sheer perseverance of our contributors who, throughout the storm, were able to keep their eye on the distant shore and stay with us on this turbulent voyage. And of course, this book is also about the personal turmoil and turbulence of what it means to be a play therapist working with troubled children, bringing together a number of experienced colleagues within the field who have been brave enough to write often deeply personal accounts of their experience of training and clinical practice. Some of the chapters challenge the unspoken therapist taboos of shame, childhood trauma, vulnerability and grief, shining a light on the more hidden areas of the human condition. Other chapters look at matters of training, supervision, self-care and illness and the importance of how, as therapists, we need to find ways to acknowledge our needs and strengthen our resilience. Clinical issues around the unconscious process and dissociation are also explored, but once again from the personal position of the play therapist, rather than the child.

The world is certainly a different place now from when we began this project, the calming waters of Moon Lake just a distant, almost surreal, abstract memory. The world has changed and of course we, as people, change too, and in a sense that is what this book is also about. Therapy is about change, process is about change and the writings in this book are all, in one way or another, about how we have felt personally and professionally challenged and changed as people and therapists. In this sense, the ethos, and indeed our hope for this book, is to honour the process of heuristic inquiry and simply allow a little space for the personhood of the play therapist to be heard. Perhaps it is the beginning of a wider conversation and if all we can do is lift up an edge of the stone and let in a little light, then so be it. Better a little light than none at all.

# Acknowledgements

We would like to thank Joanne Forshaw, our commissioning editor, and all at Routledge for their support, guidance, trust and patience along the way.

Thank you also to all our contributors, whose personal courage and resolve made this project possible, and to the children and families from whom as play therapists we learn so much.

## David

I would like to thank Elise for being part of this co-editing journey; it was not quite the one we expected. I would also like to thank Nicky and Jess, for simply being there (DLV).

## Elise

Heartfelt thanks to my co-editor, David, for all his help and support in getting this text to publication. The journey has had many twists and turns! I also want to thank my family for their unwavering support and encouragement. (EC)

Chapter 1

# 'The child is the father of the man'

## Paternal patterns of countertransference and empathy

*David Le Vay*

## Introduction

*Nathan, a forceful seven-year-old, gives me a defiant stare and tips the entire basket of objects into the sand tray, a chaotic clamour of marbles, keys, figures, stones and shells that tumble haphazardly onto the yielding sand, forming an impromptu mountain that rises dramatically from the tray like some kind of primeval lost island. The remainder spills across the floor as he tosses the basket across the room. Searching for the right words, I do my best to capture the feeling, reflecting Nathan's anger and resistance and his desperate unhappiness at feeling tricked by his father into attending this first meeting together (his father had not told him that he was coming to see me, saying that they were just going to the shops). I empathise with him; I too feel tricked and in effect we have both been set up within this first encounter by a desperate father seeking help for his troubled son. Nathan moves to sit nearer his father, grabbing handfuls of gel water beads on route that he proceeds to wrap up in tissue paper and then methodically stamp, squash and grind into the carpet, a mess of paper and crushed beads forming a victorious circle of debris around his feet.*

*"Wow, you are angry – you are really showing me how angry and cross you are. You don't want to be here right now". Nathan glowers intensely at me. His father apologises and admonishes his son for the mess he has made. "I guess you are wondering what I am going to do now" I say to Nathan. "Tell you to stop? Ask you to leave? Get angry with you? You are wondering if you really can do pretty much whatever you choose here in the playroom". Once again, he fixes me with a rebellious glint in his eye. "Yeah . . . I am testing you out" he says steadily.*

I was taken aback by such a conscious and purposeful challenge by a child in a first meeting. Another part of me thought "*yes – good for you*". Nathan felt tricked and deceived, rightly so, and consequently his capacity for trust was severely compromised. He was angry with his father and angry with me, and I did indeed feel tested by him and anxious about my capacity to meet the challenge in hand. And I also wondered about the nature of the challenge. Who is really being tested here? Myself? Nathan? His father? Perhaps all of us. But the battle lines had

DOI: 10.4324/9781003017271-1

certainly been drawn and whilst I felt daunted by the potential sessions ahead, I immediately liked Nathan very much – his energy and vitality and the directness of his communication.

After the session was over, I surveyed the debris, wondering about its meaning – the fragmented volcanic tower rising from the sand tray and spilling out of the tray and across the playroom floor like the tail of a fiery comet; and perhaps most striking of all, the congealed circular mess of crushed water beads and tissue paper, ground forcefully into the carpet around where Nathan had been sitting. Given the egg like quality of the beads, it felt like the therapeutic waters had broken – a strange birthing of sorts within this room of fathers and sons. There was something about Nathan that occupied a space within me, some-thing that I recognised from my own childhood and although the feeling was hard to place, the prevailing sense I was left with was that of sadness, anxiety and loneliness.

As I rather wearily cleared up the playroom, an end of session ritual familiar to all play therapists, I found myself thinking about both Nathan and the many other children who have passed through this space. Our therapy rooms are littered with the remains of past relationships, belonging to both the therapist and the child, the scattered figures embodied within the play, ghostly resurrections of oedipal struggles, epic battles, heroic victories and desperate defeats. Play therapists are like time travellers and the playroom like the TARDIS (always bigger on the inside) as we move back and forth in time with children, allowing their magical imagination to take us on journeys back to key developmental stages in their lives. And following Nathan's session, as I reflected upon the emotional remains of the day, the internalised presence of my own father and my experiences of early childhood somehow felt very close by. What is it about this seven-year-old boy that has touched me so deeply? How can I understand the poignant feelings that he seems to have evoked so strongly within me? Whose mess am I really clearing up?

With questions such as these in mind, my aim within this chapter is to explore the personal echoes that can become played out within our work as play therapists and the relational patterns of the unconscious process. Specifically, as a male play therapist, I am interested in my experience of paternal countertransference and how this both helps and hinders my capacity to be present and paternally empathic with the children who I am working with. To be honest, as I write these words, it feels a daunting, uncertain prospect and I am not sure where this road will lead me, but then this is a book about personal process and it is in this spirit that I embark upon this journey. Indeed, it is a little like embarking upon the therapeu-tic journey. As therapists, we are taught to tolerate uncertainty, but of course for many of the children that we are working with, change and unpredictability is all they know, and this sense of permanent impermanence also resonates powerfully with aspects of my own childhood. As the seminal author Ursula le Guinn once wrote, "the only thing that makes life possible is permanent, intolerable uncer-tainty: not knowing what comes next" (1969: 70).

## "Where the fog is thickest, begin" (Marty Rubin)

So what does come next? I am rather fearful of the permanence of the printed word; the notion of writing as an indelible act of finality and the sense of something becoming fixed, like a mark on paper; very different, for example, from the ephemeral, transient nature of children's play or the passing image in a sand tray. And at the heart of this struggle is finding a comfortable setting on my personal filter, the extent to which I move my internal slider between the opposing points of transparency and opaqueness and make myself visible within the words of this chapter. To write about paternal empathy and countertransference within a context of personal process requires, by definition, an act of introspection and self-examination regarding my own experience of both childhood and fatherhood and all that this means and within this context I am struck by the notion of the indelible, beyond the printed word. We are all, in one way or another, left marked by our relational experiences throughout the passage of our lives. We are shaped, sculpted, carved and patterned by the prevailing winds of experience that course through time, blowing through the years. Wherever we go, there we are.

When I think of countertransference I think of *patterns of expectation* – deeply embedded unconscious patterns of relating that we carry with us, for better or worse, and which are often conjured unexpectedly into existence through the course of the therapeutic encounter. We cannot, and indeed should not, remove ourselves from this encounter; it is after all an interaction – a relationship. Play therapy is a relational process and this requires, by definition, the active use of self (Le Vay, 2016) as an authentic and congruent agent for change, for both the play therapist and the child. As Jung (1933) suggests, the therapeutic encounter is akin to the interaction between two chemical substances; if there is a reaction, then both are transformed and this is just as it should be. This relational lens explicitly acknowledges the interactive nature of the therapeutic process in the sense that there is an intersubjective overlap between the play therapist and the child. More though than just an overlap, this is more about a process of becoming emotionally joined, intertwined, often entangled, as the creative potential of the play therapy space is filled with the ethereal presence of past relationships, revitalised and magically brought to life.

The fog is indeed thickest when I reflect upon my early years and the relationship with my own father. Wordsworth (1994) wrote that "*the child is father of the man*" and I am deeply conscious of how much my adult years have been shaped by my early, formative childhood experiences. My father was in many ways a brilliant man: orthopaedic surgeon, academic, writer, musician, multi-linguist and translator; indeed, something of the classic polymath. But for all that, he was not a great father. He lived throughout his life with severe mental health difficulties, and whilst as a young child I can recall periods of delightful charisma, charm and playfulness (wonderful qualities for a father), he was more often than not distant, unpredictable, hyper-critical, frightening and often emotionally abusive. During my early childhood years, I rode the storm, a little like a surfer, learning when to pick out and ride the exciting high rollers and when to avoid the more destructive, darker, turbulent seas. But during my teenage years, to stay for a moment with the metaphor, the storm became too great and I was wiped out by one too many crashing waves and so retreated to the deeper, half-lit waters of adolescence. Indeed, it was only later on, in my twenties, that I became fully aware of the nature and meaning of his diagnosis and could begin to understand his behaviour, and our relationship, within a wider mental health context.

But as a young child there is no context, just subjective experience and unspoken questions. Does he hate me? Is it my fault? What have I done wrong? Am I safe? Why is my mother crying? Throughout childhood I desperately sought my father's approval, which never came, and learned from an early age that there was always going to be a part of me that would never, as Winnicott (1953) might say, be "*good enough*". Ironically, after my father died, we discovered amongst his many documents an unpublished alternative version of his autobiography in which he wrote, amongst other things, about his experience of engaging in psychoanalysis over many years, which at one point included a consultation with Winnicott himself. My father wrote of this encounter:

> He (Winnicott) sat opposite me, put his hand over his eyes – not the usual form – and did more for me in an hour than anyone else in a year. He began by saying, "you know, I had the feeling that you might be coming for me with a gun" – quite amazing intuition since this had been exactly my own visual imagining. He also told me that I had to be my own father, having denied (or been denied) a loving paternal relationship. That too was exactly right and no-one had ever said it before.
>
> (A.D. Le Vay, 1970: 120)

It seemed that Winnicott had quickly got to the heart of my father's rage and paternal deprivation and so in turn, in a strange kind of way, he has also helped me to understand something about my relationship with my own father and the absence of any kind of paternal empathy when I was a young child. There were also many times when, like Winnicott, I thought my father might be "coming for me with a gun", so to speak. These scripts are strong, generational and deeply embedded within our unconscious. When he was alive, my father never spoke of his own childhood; it was the one "book" of his that remained firmly closed, and so the discovery after his death of his many years of psychoanalysis and his apparent search to find some kind of truth or resolution within his troubled past had a profound impact upon me. So it turns out that my father never felt "*good enough*" either, and the story he left behind about his own early years (left perhaps for his children to find) described a troubled relationship with his own father, who was harsh, critical and punitive.

I share this story because it is an important part of who I am as a person and as a therapist. The child is indeed the father of the man and without knowing it, I have in a sense also had to take Winnicott's advice to "be my own father" and find ways to integrate the good with the bad, reject the ugly and fill in the spaces in between. This has been a long journey and took many years of personal reflection and exploration through training, personal therapy, supervision and clinical practice. And of course, it has led me to reflect much upon my own experience of parenthood, not so much being my own father but being a new, different kind of father. On our path to becoming and being a therapist, I would suggest that we do need to begin where the fog is thickest, to feel our way ahead as we gradually develop a sense of the particular contours that shape and form our internal landscape and that help us to navigate a way forward.

## Some reflections on countertransference and play therapy

Whilst there is significant acknowledgement of the role of the unconscious process within child centred play therapy (CCPT), little has been written specifically about the role of countertransference, which is perhaps due in part to the Rogerian (Rogers 1951) theoretical orientation of CCPT and the fact that ideas of transference and countertransference are considered less important, or perhaps given less weight, within a humanistic therapeutic tradition that places more emphasis on the current "here and now" nature of the therapeutic relationship. That said, play therapy owes much to the early psychodynamic, analytic work of people like Anna Freud (1927), Klein (1932) Lowenfeld (1935) and of course Winnicott (1971) who all in their own way recognised the symbolic, unconscious and primarily non-verbal nature (and value) of children's play.

An understanding of countertransference begins, as ever, with Freud, who viewed it mainly as a negative phenomenon: a personal problem of the analyst that threatened to contaminate the transference from the "patient". Freud described countertransference as something "arising in the physician as a result of the patient's influence on his (the physician's) unconscious feeling" (1910: 144) and in this sense, it was understood as a phenomenon arising as a direct response/reaction to the patient's transference and something to be "mastered" and managed, a potential hindrance to the analytic process. But certainly, moving on from these early origins, there has been a developing, evolving conceptual understanding and acknowledgement of countertransference as a valuable and intrinsic aspect of the therapeutic process. More than just a reaction to the client's unconscious transferential communication, countertransference is now understood within a much wider relational field, that is as the more generic unconscious influence of the therapist's past relational experiences upon the therapeutic process. So more broadly speaking, this might include all of the therapist's thoughts, feelings and behaviours, both conscious and unconscious, that impact upon or influence the process. This might indeed be in response to the client's issues but alternatively might be rooted within the therapist's own unresolved internal conflicts and early relational experiences.

In relation to CCPT with young children, I would suggest that countertransference responses and reactions can be particularly complex and intense. There is a powerful, dynamic immediacy to children's therapeutic play, which is not mediated, moderated or filtered by the more cognitive verbal process. Clearly, there is an emotional and aesthetic distance facilitated via the metaphoric and symbolic nature of the play, more so I would suggest for the child than the therapist, although emotional distance is experienced to a greater or lesser extent depending upon the nature of the play. Through the course of a child's dramatic play in particular, we often find ourselves inhabiting the role of the parent, child, sibling and more often than not, victim or persecutor. Our countertransference responses to the child's play communication will inevitably be both influenced and informed by the intersubjective nature of the therapeutic encounter and the complex psychodynamic and more intrasubjective nature of personal experience that intrinsically contributes to our sense of self, for example our experiences of loss, bereavement, separation, trauma and our broader personal associations and memories of early childhood. In this sense, our responses are the result of the interplay between the external and the internal. We might find ourselves over-identifying with the child, or seeking to distance ourselves from them, or feeling critical, nurturing, punitive or over-protective and so our therapeutic boundaries might become distorted, blurred or pulled out of shape – a strong indication of the influence and impact of countertransference upon the therapeutic process.

So, our personal responses are many, varied and multi-layered and as Gil and Rubin (2005) suggest, the rather traditional and linear "cause-and-effect" conceptualisation of countertransference as a "reciprocal relationship between the client's transference and the therapist's unconscious" (2005: 89) is perhaps limited and oversimplified. Our conscious and unconscious countertransference responses communicate much about both the child's and our own internal worlds; therein lies the entanglement, but beyond that our responses can also be key to an awareness of (and insight into) the wider systemic context of the child's world. I worked for many years with highly traumatised looked-after children who were displaying harmful sexual behaviour, and was often struck by the intense feelings generated through the work. The fear, disgust, anxiety and often complex victim/perpetrator dynamics became enacted, mirrored and played out by the professional network and family system – a distorted reflection of the child's fragmented and traumatised inner world. Perhaps then, beyond the relationships between child and therapist, we need to be mindful of the wider systemic nature (and organisational impact) of countertransference reactions. As Britton suggests, "that the more primitive mechanisms and defences against anxiety are being used the more is every professional contact likely to become a scene for action and for the professional to yield . . . to re-enact an unconscious situation" (Britton, 1995: 52).

## Countertransference and paternal empathy

The relationship between countertransference and empathy and how we manage these feelings is an important part of this discussion, specifically, how as play therapists we are able to maintain a congruent, authentic and empathic response to children in the face of the often powerfully projective nature of the therapeutic process and play content. As said, the therapeutic relationship is one of intersubjectivity, the space in between the subjective worlds of the child and the therapist – the relationship between self and other. As Benjamin (1990) suggests, the process of discovering and recognising the other as "subject" creates an experience of our own subjectivity, a sense of mutual recognition. It this sense of mutual recognition that evokes the essence of empathy, defined by Clark (1980) as that "unique capacity of the human being to feel the experiences, needs, aspirations, frustrations, sorrows, joys, anxieties, hurt or hunger as if they were his or her own" (1980: 190). This empathic sense of experiencing something as if it were our own clearly presents significant challenges when working with highly traumatised children. It requires an act of "stepping into" the child's world and all that this means – a world that is often filled with fear, rage, shame, distrust and anxiety. Equally important is the act of "stepping out" and being mindful of the extent in which we can become over-immersed in the child's world. For these children, interpersonal boundaries (their own intersubjective experience) have been abusive, distorted, shapeless, terrifying and unpredictable. Creating a therapeutic relationship with these children, emotionally connecting with their internal worlds, can be a daunting and at times disturbing experience that can challenge one's capacity to remain attuned and empathic.

*Nathan had been dictating a story to me about two armies involved in a violent bloody battle, when he paused and said he wanted to take the story home after his session. I explained, as I had before, that I would keep everything safe for him in his box and that he could then decide what to take home when we have our final session together.*

N  *That's a stupid rule – I want to take it home today.*
T  *You think it is a stupid rule? Well, it is a play therapy rule – but it sounds like you think some rules are stupid?*
N  *You only have that rule for me*
T  *No, it is the same rule for everyone I see*
N  *(Getting angry) So where all the other boxes? It's just my rule – I want to take it today.*
T  *Rules feel unfair sometimes.*
N  *I am going to stop coming to stupid play therapy unless I can take it home.*
T  *Wow, you are cross. Well, that would be a shame. I would miss you. I hope you keep coming to your sessions.*
N  *(Pleading) Please let me take it.*

*I am aware of feeling mean, withholding and punitive. I find myself internally questioning the rule. Is it stupid? I feel myself wavering – maybe I should just let him have what he wants? Will it really matter?*

T  *So what would you do with your story if you took it home?*
N  *I would read to Amy (younger sister) and scare her with it.*

> T   Well, it is a scary story – about people fighting and hurting and killing each
>      other. I don't think it would be a good idea to scare Amy with it, do you? It
>      is important for me to keep your things safe here – for me to look after the
>      scary stuff.
> N   Why are you being so mean to me?

*Am I the bully now I wonder? The punitive father? Nathan goes through a reper-
toire of strategies to try and get his way. He makes a clearly well-rehearsed imp-
ish, endearing facial expression.*

> T   Ah . . . so is that the face you use when you want to get your way?
> N   Yes.
> T   And does it usually work?
> N   Yes, always.
> T   Well, I am afraid your story stays in your box here.

*Nathan gets angrier. I am sitting on the floor and he stands over me and pretends
to hit and punch me, trying to make me flinch.*

> N   There, I saw you – I saw your eyes move.
> T   You want to frighten me – because you can't get what you want?
> T   I wonder what happens at school with your friends when you can't get your
>      way.
> N   They are frightened of me.
> T   Ah, I see. So, you try and frighten them if you can't get your way.

*I briefly make a link to the bullying at school that led to him being initially referred
for play therapy, about the frightening things that have happened to him, but he
tells me to stop talking, shuts me up and makes a big play of ignoring anything
I say by exaggeratingly mocking me. I am aware of feeling annoyed and irritated
with Nathan. There is a forceful sense of entitlement about him that is unlikeable,
and I am aware of wanting the session to end. I struggle to hold onto any kind of
emotional empathy, as if a drawbridge has been suddenly pulled up from between
us and underneath all this, I experience a fleeting but deep feeling of humiliation,
shame perhaps, that seems to come from an entirely different place.*

*After the session has ended and Nathan has left, without his story, I try to make
sense of what happened, but it feels vague and intangible and hard to get hold
of. Between the written words of war hastily scribbled on the embattled piece
of paper that lies forlornly beside the sand tray, it is clear that another story
has been told here. This small child's transference is a communication perhaps
about fathers who can feel harsh, punitive and critical, a dramatic enactment of
Nathan's narrated story about two armies engaged in violent battle. And what of
the countertransference? In part, I think my feelings communicated something
about how Nathan is at times experienced by his own father, a direct reaction to*

*his transference which in turn helped me understand something of the pattern of*
*relating played out between them. But beyond that lies something else; something*
*that belongs more to myself and my own paternal story. Nathan's desperate need*
*for approval and his quicksilver flight into anxious retreat triggered something*
*deeply imprinted within my own psyche, a feeling which I meet briefly before*
*looking away, avoidant and defended – a gaze averted, such is the experience of*
*childhood shame.*

And this is where the entanglement lies: the complexity of countertransference. My own deeply felt personal narrative around the absence of paternal empathy and a father who could be withholding and persecutory seeps and leaks into the shared intersubjective space of the session, an osmotic merging of sorts, and I find myself struggling to untangle the knotted threads to see which end belongs where and with whom. It is critical then that as play therapists we are ever mindful of our personal stories and emotional responses, both conscious and unconscious, evoked by the child. And perhaps too, it is important to acknowledge that there will be times when we feel less able to be fully present, attuned and empathic. Indeed, to be fully congruent at all times is perhaps more of a therapeutic aspiration than a reality. Working therapeutically with children can present very particular and unique countertransference challenges for the play therapist. As Brandell (1992) suggests, there are various factors that might contribute towards these challenges. Unlike adults, children lack the conscious motivation or indeed choice regarding treatment. They are also more "action oriented", that is, they engage through the immediacy of play and are easily frustrated and "inherently regressive" (1992: 90). In this sense, children have been described as potential countertransference tinderboxes (Gabel & Bemporad, 1994), in many ways an apt description that captures something about the often emotionally volatile nature of working with troubled children.

## Intersubjectivity and the liminal space within play therapy

As discussed, much of our work as play therapists takes place in the world of the "as if", the magical symbolic space that sits somewhere in between fantasy and reality in which the child's active imagination and their innate playful creativity, held within the safety of the therapeutic relationship, enable a process of transformation and healing to occur. The relationship of course is key and, in many ways, this is analogous to Winnicott's (1971) concept of the potential space, the intersubjective psychic field between the parent and the infant, which allows for safe playful exploration whilst still feeling connected: to be able to play in the containing presence of another. As Winnicott states

> [T]he potential space between baby and mother, between child and family, between individual and society or the world, depends on experience

(derived from play) which leads to trust. It can be looked upon as sacred to the individual in that it is here that the individual experiences creative living.

(1971: 103)

Within the creative potentiality of the play therapy space, children will play out, enact, re-enact and return to key development stages and ages in their lives, often places of unmet need or trauma, and this will invariably engender powerful feelings within the therapist around significant areas of need or conflict within their own developmental experience.

Drawing upon this analogy between the therapist and the parent, Winnicott, in his paper "Hate in the Countertransference", suggests that the analyst needs to "display all of the patience and tolerance and reliability of a mother devoted to her infant . . . and has to seem to want to give what is really only given because of the patient's needs" (1994: 356). This then again evokes the parallel between the therapeutic relationship and the interpersonal space between infant and care-giver and is evocative of the embodied sensation of often very primal need (hunger perhaps?) experienced by abused and neglected children and the importance of separating out which need belongs where and to whom. Nathan, with his challenging, persecutory and sometimes aggressive behaviour, was communicating an unconscious need – for safety, predictability and limits within which he could feel emotionally held and contained. As therapists we need to be alert to the feeling beneath the behaviour and to the need beneath the feeling, in the same sense, as Winnicott suggests, the primary carer needs to be attentive to the primary needs of the infant.

Beyond Winnicott, developing theory and evidence from attachment studies, neuroscience and developmental psychology, amongst others, continues to inform our work as therapists and places, I would suggest, a much greater emphasis upon the intersubjective nature of the therapeutic relationship as well as contributing to a developing and perhaps more contemporary understanding of the role of transference and countertransference. Valerio (2017) emphasises the "paradigmatic shift" within contemporary psychotherapy towards the body over mind and an understanding of countertransference more in terms of an embodied, affective state. They suggest that "countertransference communications are experienced affectively, by the therapist, feeling states or mood alteration, but often as a bodily reaction" (2017: 29). This is important; countertransference is by definition a largely unconscious process and hence lies imperceptibly beyond our conscious awareness – the known unknown, so to speak. But if we are able to understand countertransference as an embodied, affective communication, it means that our physical, embodied and felt responses can provide valuable clues to our own and the child's unconscious process and the feelings engendered therein. Feeling tired, sick, bored, excited, aroused or perhaps vicarious somatic expressions of traumatic pain in the form of stomach aches or headaches are all important responses to be monitored and explored within personal therapy or clinical supervision and which can provide valuable insight into the child's internal world and what is being communicated within the therapeutic process. Interestingly, and aptly within this context of affective unconscious communication, Diamond and Valerio conceptualise this experience of a felt response to the client's trauma as a form of "counterdissociation", suggesting that

> It is as if the analyst's body mirrors theirs in cutting off from feelings which exist in the patient, yet without narrative and verbal recall of events. The thing about embodied countertransference reactions is that the therapist will also have periods of unawareness. The hope is to have enough active engagement with one's own unconscious process to rapidly bring this into greater awareness so that it can be worked with in the consulting room.
>
> (Valerio, 2017: 28)

Valerio (2017), in her seminal volume on countertransference within therapeutic practice, also talks of the "liminal zone" within therapeutic work (Valerio, 2017), the "space in-between" so inherent within the notion of the intersubjective. Deriving from the Latin word *limes*, meaning "threshold", we can think of the liminal space as place of transition, change and potentiality. It is a place betwixt and between; unknowable, ambiguous and unpredictable and for therapists it may indeed occupy a place on the edge of comfort – a place where, some might suggest, much of the important therapeutic work gets done. Within anthropology, we can think of liminal space within a ritualistic context, sacred even, both mythic and mystic, and in this sense, it is important to consider parallels with the ritualistic nature of the play therapy process. CCPT takes place at a given time within a given place and within a given form of therapeutic limits and boundaries. In terms of delivery, it is both sequential and prescribed in nature, hence providing both physical and psychological structure and form that enables the child to engage creatively through play.

Of course, within the child centred play therapy process itself, the child has the freedom and autonomy to choose how to play, and again ritualistic patterns of play often emerge, for example within physical and vocal gesture, repeated patterns of play behaviour, movement or activity. A very traumatised and dissociative child I worked with for many months would routinely start each session by going to the sand tray and gently smoothing the sand with her hands as she hummed quietly to herself. It was her "sand song" and the way of self-regulating that over time became something of a ritual that enabled her to transition into the play therapy space. The notion of liminal space – the "threshold" – applies also to the nature of play itself. Children's play takes place on the margins of reality, a place between the symbolic and the real – under a table, in a box, in a treehouse, in the corner. As A. A. Milne captured so well in his poem "Halfway Down", children's imagination occupies a transient space between worlds – "all sorts of funny thoughts run around my head, it isn't really anywhere, it's somewhere else instead" (1934: 81).

And in terms of transference and countertransference, there is the liminal zone between the conscious and the unconscious, like the transitional area of sandy beach between ocean and land, the intimate edge (Ehrenberg, 1974) between self and other, where we variously meet, retreat, connect, disconnect and ebb and flow throughout the course of the therapeutic encounter. It is an area of overlay and entwinement, often surprising, as the turbulent waters of the unconscious bring up long-lost objects, forgotten fragments of shell and stone, raised from the depths and thrown into sharp relief as they lay deposited and revealed upon the shimmering sands of conscious awareness. As therapists, we are all familiar with the experience of reverie, that dreamy, dissociative state of whimsical musing and mindful wandering (and indeed wondering) as we seek to both sense and make sense of what is happening in the child's mind, as well as our own. It is a threshold of sorts, a fertile place for the creative imagination and in relation to the unconscious process, deeply evocative.

*Nathan brings some football cards with him that he likes to collect in albums. He goes about making an album for me and then wants to give me some of his spare cards that he does not need. There is a sense of us being the same – joined in shared endeavour. He says I should take the picture album home just as he will take his home. There is an emotional intimacy within the play and I feel warmly towards Nathan and experience a deep sense of connection that feels reminiscent of a sibling relationship, more fraternal than paternal. I recall as a child, Nathan's age, collecting cards just like him. There is a comfort in collecting; the ordering, sequencing, sharing and playful playground bartering as cards are exchanged like precious currency. Or collecting stamps with my brothers – carefully sticking them down with specially hinged pieces of gummed paper. For a moment I feel transported back to my seven-year-old self and am surprised by the sudden and unexpected emergence of these childhood remembrances. It is an odd moment of collecting and recollecting. I wonder what this might mean. What it might be communicating about Nathan's needs; the lone son within a fractious, troubled family, expressing a need to feel close, or simply a feeling of sameness? There is an intense sense of loss and longing here too, mutual perhaps: for myself an expression of what I once had and for Nathan for what he most desires. The countertransference brings with it a deep sense of intimate empathy in contrast to previous sessions wherein I felt pushed away, distant and disconnected. As I sit and play with Nathan I feel delicately poised upon the liminal threshold between self and other. As Benjamin (1990) suggests, this quality of intersubjectivity involves the capacity to hold the tension between relating to the other as both object and subject – the internal and the external. But it is a delicate, temporal moment of closeness. Nathan struggles to make the album just as he wants it to be. He asks for help but I cannot get it right either. He gets anxious, frustrated, impatient and angry. The paper rips, the stapler does not staple, the cards do not fit properly and suddenly his world collapses and I lose him again, along with my childhood remembrances. Such are our fragile worlds.*

Inevitably, working therapeutically with young children brings us into contact with our own early experiences and associations. Ultimately, this kind of work cannot help but stimulate and revive memories of our own childhood, within which we become entwined and entangled with the child's own experience. As Bonovitz (2009) questions, do these personal remembrances remain located within our own private, internalised dialogue, separate from the child? Or should we think of them as existing within the relational arena of the unconscious process? Bonovitz goes onto to suggest:

> The revival of these childhood recollections in the analyst is not necessarily a barrier or sign of pathology as previously held, but rather in some cases is a vital resource that may potentially deepen and facilitate analytic work. The focus here is on those situations when the unexpected arrival of the analyst's childhood in the playroom may be used to elucidate the transference/countertransference field.
>
> (2009: 236)

There are then some particular qualities of working therapeutically with young children that contribute to the potential intensity of our unconscious responses. Feelings around parental responsibility and protectiveness will always be close by, as will be the dynamics of power and vulnerability, no less evident than in the manifest difference in physical size – the "big" therapist and the "little" child. A child hides behind a chair, awaiting with keen anticipation the joy of being found, or engages in an epic battle between good and evil – sword at the ready. Or a hand is buried in the sand tray and slowly uncovered in a poignant moment of self-discovery. There is an intimacy to these moments that can bring with them the momentary revival of our own childhoods, often sudden and unexpected visitors in the playroom. At various times, we might love or hate or indeed feel indifferent to the children whom we are working with, feelings revealed within the countertransference, but the nature of working with children brings intensity to these feelings that is very different from working with adults. Ultimately, it is about the play relationship wherein we are connecting through action, sound, movement, gesture and affect; and through object play, role-play or sensory engagement. In this sense the way we experience and indeed communicate our countertransference responses is in contrast to the more cognitive, verbal nature of working with adults. This again brings us back to the embodied quality of the unconscious process when working with children and the physicality of the relationship, often communicated very powerfully and directly.

*Nathan is in role as sheriff and I am assigned the role of a "bad robber" who has stolen money from the bank. The sheriff catches the robber and shoots and kills him, a sequence repeated by Nathan several times as he rewinds and replays the scene with some intensity. The robber is resurrected and placed in jail, which becomes a lion's den. Nathan becomes the lion and rips great chunks of flesh from the robber. As I move in and out of role, allowing Nathan to direct the action, various scenes in which the robber is caught and punished are enacted with a visceral enthusiasm. I wonder aloud what the robber might have done to deserve such punishment. The robber is placed in a bear pit and Nathan is the bear, ripping the robber to shreds with his teeth and claws. The robber is then moved into a tiger den where the robber is eaten – his eyes pulled out, his body slashed and then finally decapitated. The robber is then transferred to prison where he is cruci-fied – the sheriff hammering the nails into the robber's hands and feet and then slitting his stomach open. I wonder how much more of this sadistic punishment I can take and it is a relief when I tell Nathan he has just five minutes of the ses-sion left. He looks at me intently and says "okay, well, I will just carry on killing you for five more minutes".*

*Afterwards I feel exhausted and emotionally drained. I wonder about my expe-riences of helplessness in the session – of feeling victimised, humiliated and exposed. I am unsure and self-critical about my responses to Nathan in the imme-diacy of the play and the aftermath of the session. Did I do enough? Say enough? Should I have intervened in some way? How could I have responded differently? Should I have told him to stop? I wonder about Nathan's father and of his time in military service and what this might have involved. And then I find myself think-ing about my own father and his behaviour towards me as a young child that was often shaming and demeaning, and my own powerlessness to make it stop. I wonder if I am over-identifying with Nathan, itself a possible indication of the countertransference. Certainly, Nathan has kept true to his challenge laid down in our first meeting – that he will test me out.*

## Reflections on the management of countertransference

Countertransference then serves to deepen and enrich our understanding of both the child's and our own emotional lives, our internal landscape. The central question is: why am I feeling like this and what does this communicate about the child's and my own relational, intersubjective world? Far from Freud's notion of countertransference as a contamination of the therapeutic process, it could instead be seen as an inherent expression of selfhood and both a recogni-tion of all that we bring to the relationship and an acknowledgement that aspects of our own history will inevitably emerge during the course of the therapeutic encounter. That said, it is important that as therapists we are mindful enough to be able to monitor, attend and be alert to the personal feelings evoked with the work. By definition, working with troubled children will evoke troubled feel-ings, often in relation to our own areas of unmet need, unresolved conflict and those key developmental stages in our personal history that remain marked in time, recorded or collected like football cards or stamps in life's rich album of remembrance.

The unconscious has a habit of sneaking up upon us, catching us off-guard and boundaries can all too easily become distorted and pulled out of shape. The unconscious is by nature largely indiscernible and so we need to be alert to the clues and cues in the work that might be indicators of the unconscious process at play. There are children we might idealise, demonise or have fantasies about rescuing. There may be feelings of love, hate, envy, avoidance and detachment and whilst I am unsure of the value in thinking about countertransference in positive or negative terms (more simply as a communication), it can clearly impact the therapeutic process detrimentally and potentially affect the outcome of the work, for example having protective feelings towards a child and critical feelings towards the parents.

So the recognition and management of countertransference are important. This demands a level of self-awareness and personal reflexivity and a willingness to engage openly in the support processes of clinical supervision and personal therapy. Research into countertransference amongst play therapists (Metcalfe, 2003) also highlighted the importance of rigorous clinical training and a strong theoretical foundation in effectively managing countertransference feelings. Gil (2005) in her paper on Countertransference Play suggests how creative arts and play-based clinical supervision can be utilised to enable practitioners to explore potential issues of countertransference within their work. Specifically, Gil argues that there is value in therapists engaging in strategies that are "consistent with the mode of treatment they typically use with their clients, namely, play therapy" (2005: 92). Certainly, in my experience, creative clinical supervision that parallels the symbolic process of play therapy and activates a more non-verbal, unconscious process of exploring client material can be both effective and helpful in the recognition of countertransference feelings. For example, it might be creating a sand tray to portray how we experience working with a particular child, or an image on paper or shape sculpted out of modelling material to embody our felt responses to the session material. Reflective writing might be helpful for some. Whatever form it might take, these processes can help the intangible become tangible – to see a way through the fog that can all too easily cloud our awareness and judgement.

## Conclusion

As stated, it was with a sense of some trepidation that I embarked upon the process of writing this chapter, not knowing quite where it might lead, where it might end and the extent to which I make myself visible within the words. There is a tension here, between withholding and disclosure, and indeed this is a tension that we all experience as therapists as we strive to find a balance between self and other, to find a position within our work that feels congruent and authentic. Whether I have achieved this balance remains to be seen although on a personal level, this exploration of paternal countertransference and empathy has been a helpful process and led to a level of reflection upon my own story around becoming and being a therapist. The child is indeed the father of the man, and the mother of the woman, but beyond this Wordsworth's short poem captures the wonder of childhood and perhaps something about how as adults we need to hold on this sense of wonder. It is a valuable resource, drawn from the deep well of childhood remembrance, that sustains us through the course of our often very challenging work with troubled children.

I have also found myself reflecting upon the extent to which the children we work with, children like Nathan, can teach us about ourselves. I would even go as far as to say that if we ever feel that we have no more to learn from the children we are working with, then it may be time to hang up our therapist hat, whatever that might look like. Nathan of course has been anonymised, pseudonymised and disguised in general; he is a composite of sorts. But to him, and the other children who have contributed to the formation of this chapter through the magical creativity of their play, I am eternally grateful.

## References

Benjamin, J. (1990) *Recognition and Destruction: An Outline of Intersubjectivity*. In: Mitchell, S. A. & Aron, L. (eds.) *Relational Psychoanalysis: The Emergence of a Tradition* (pp. 181–211). Hillsdale, NJ: The Analytic Press.

Bonovitz, C. (2009) Countertransference in Child Psychoanalytic Psychotherapy: The Emergence of the Analyst's Childhood. *Psychoanalytic Psychology*, 26(3), pp. 235–245.

Brandell, J. R. (1992) *Countertransference in Psychotherapy With Children and Adolescents*. Northvale, NJ: Jason Aronson.

Britton, R. (1995) Re-Enactment as an Unwitting Professional Response to Family Dynamics'. In: Bower, M. (ed.) *Psychoanalytic Ideas for Child and Family Social Work*. London: Routledge.

Clark, K. B. (1980) Empathy: A Neglected Topic in Psychological Research. *American Psychologist*, 35, pp. 187–190.

Ehrenberg, D. (1974) The Intimate Edge in Therapeutic Relatedness. *Contemporary Psychoanalysis*, 10, pp. 423–437.

Freud, A. (1927) Introduction to the Technique of Child Analysis. In: *The Writings of Anna Freud*. New York: International Universities Press, 1974.

Freud, S. (ed. & trans. Strachey, J. 1910) *The Future Prospects of Psychoanalytic Therapy. The Standard Edition of the Complete Psychological Works of Sigmund Freud* (vol. 11, pp. 144–145). London: Hogarth.

Gabel, S. & Bemporad, J. (1994) Variations in Countertransference Reactions in Psychotherapy With Children. *American Journal of Psychiatry*, 48(1), pp. 111–120.

Gil, E. & Rubin, L. (2005) Countertransference Play: Informing and Enhancing Therapist Self Awareness Through Play. *International Journal of Play Therapy*, 14(2), pp. 87–102.

Jung, C. (1933) *Modern Man in Search of a Soul*. London: Routledge.

Klein, M. (1932) *The Psycho-Analysis of Children*. London: The Hogarth Press and the Institute of Psycho-Analysis.

Lowenfeld, M. (1935) *Play in Childhood*. New York: Mac Keith Press Distributed by Cambridge University Press, 1991 (Originally published in 1935).

Le Guin, U. K. (1969) *The Left Hand of Darkness*. New York: Penguin.

Le Vay, A. D. (1970) Unpublished Autobiography.

Le Vay, D. (2016) To Be or Not to Be? The Therapeutic Use of Self Within Child Centred Play Therapy. In: Le Vay, D. & Cuschieri, E. (eds.) *Challenges in the Theory and Practice of Play Therapy*. London: Routledge.

Metcalfe, L. M. (2003) Countertransference Among Play Therapists: Implications for Therapist Development and Supervision. *International Journal of Play Therapy*, 12(2), pp. 31–48.

Milne, A. A. (1934) *When We Were Very Young*. London: Methuen.

Rogers, C. R. (1951) *Client-Centred Therapy*. Boston, MA: Houghton Mifflin.

Rubin, M. (no date) *Goodreads*. Available at: www.goodreads.com/ (Accessed: 15 November 2019).

Valerio, P. (2017) *Introduction to Countertransference in Therapeutic Practice: A Myriad of Mirrors*. London: Routledge.

Winnicott, D. W. (1994) Hate in the Countertransference. *Journal of Psychotherapy Practice and Research*, 3(4), 1994, pp. 348–356.

Winnicott, D. W. (1953) Transitional Objects and Transitional Phenomena: A Study of the First Not-Me Possession. *International Journal of Psychoanalysis*, 34(2), pp. 89–97.

Winnicott, D. W. (1971) *Playing and Reality*. London: Routledge.

Wordsworth, W. (1994) *The Collected Poems of William Wordsworth*. Herts: Wordsworth Editions. New Edition.

# Chapter 2

# Thresholds and transitions

## From trainee to therapist and trainer

*Elise Cuschieri*

As I sit down to write the introduction to this chapter, a myriad of memories, thoughts and feelings come flooding in: I am transported back to an Airbus A359 and the inception of this book when David (Le Vay, co-editor of this volume) and I were flying back to the United Kingdom from a conference in China. The conference was about play in its widest sense: from education and therapy to gaming and architecture. I came away feeling stimulated, enthusiastic and with a new energy to be creative. Flying over the Gobi Desert, David and I talked about play and play therapy, about our careers and our hopes for the future of play therapy in the United Kingdom. We discussed the role of the therapist and acknowledged, not for the first time, the dearth of literature about the experience of play therapy from the play therapist's personal perspective. We both articulated the need for a follow-up text to the first book that we had edited together. It was then that our second book, this volume, was conceived.

Since first starting work on this chapter sometime in early 2019, the months have flown by and events have changed rapidly. As I write this draft, we are emerging from our third national lockdown in March 2021 – – a very different world to that of October 2018 when David and I travelled back from China. Global events, apparently originating by some curious quirk in China, have forced the international community to stop in its tracks over the past 12 months and, along with everyone else, my life has changed. On a professional level, together with colleagues, we have adapted and adjusted both our teaching and our play therapy practice: the need to find solutions to, initially, insurmountable obstacles has challenged all of us and, for all of us, our work has evolved and changed. The creative juices stimulated in China in 2018 have certainly been put to the test.

Perhaps not unsurprisingly, my focus for this chapter has also evolved and changed. I started out intending to write a follow-up to my first chapter where I had articulated some thoughts and perspectives on the phenomenon of therapist self-doubt. However, over the past months, I have given much thought to the experience of our trainees on the MA Play Therapy programme as well as to play therapy practice and teaching. I decided it seemed relevant to explore these different but interrelated roles of trainee and therapist from my personal experience,

DOI: 10.4324/9781003017271-2

and also from my perspective as trainer, considering some of the key experiences and processes that inform and link them together.

## Crossing the threshold: from teacher to therapy trainee

I had a clear plan when I applied for play therapy training in the United Kingdom. At the time, I was still living in Malta where I was born and grew up. I would go to the United Kingdom, do the training and return home to set up play therapy. Back in the late 1990s, there was a dearth of services for children needing emotional support and I was determined to change that. My then partner had recently set up an independent therapy practice for adults. It had an additional small adjoining room with a sink – perfect for working with children, or so I thought. At that point, I did not appreciate just how loud play therapy sessions can get. My imagination ran ahead of me: the room was ready; the children needing emotional support were certainly "out there". I just needed to qualify. I entered the training believing that focused hard work would see me through and that I would emerge the other end a confident and competent play therapist, ready to take on the world, or at least tiny Malta.

That was in the early 2000s. I am still living in the United Kingdom. Things did not quite go according to plan.

The early days, weeks and months of starting training tested me – not just stepping over the threshold into the sudden immersion of a therapy training that would often feel like I was being turned inside out but also the challenges of setting up a new life in a country which, whilst not completely foreign to me due to strong familial links, was nevertheless a place I had not lived in. Even setting up a bank account in the years before Malta joined the EU was complex. But as the days and weeks went by, I felt invigorated, stimulated and also challenged; and one of the first challenges was giving myself permission to engage in a process that would very quickly make me question so many aspects of myself and my life. I was surprised by this and therein lay the crux of it: at the point of applying for the training, I did not really expect to be challenged so intensely. I thought I was reasonably self-aware, I had 20-odd years of working with children behind me and I had continued to be engaged in higher education studies. I believed I had the skills needed to support children who had experienced difficult life events. It was not overconfidence but it was a lack of understanding of what training to be a therapist actually involved. I had done the standard pre-course reading: Axline's Dibs (Axline, 1990) and Play Therapy (Axline, 1989), and had been in personal therapy before moving to the United Kingdom. I thought I was prepared for the work ahead but had definitely underestimated the work involved, on both personal and academic levels.

To engage in the training process in a genuine manner, trainees are invited to be open and honest with themselves and with others on the training, both training peers and trainers. When I joined my training group, I was looking forward to learning with a group of strangers. After living in Malta for over three decades, coming to the anonymity of London was liberating. For readers unfamiliar with Malta, it is a tiny independent island state situated in the Mediterranean Sea, with Italy to the north and Tunisia to the east. It has a population of around 500,000 and is 316 km², making it the tenth smallest country in the world, and giving it the sobering claim of being the fourth most densely populated sovereign country in the world (Wikipedia Contributors, 2019). The common perception with small places that everyone knows everyone else is not too far from the truth in Malta so setting up home in multicultural London felt exciting and refreshing.

My training group and I quickly found ourselves engaged in a learning process that was thought-provoking and demanding. I had not anticipated just how exposing experiential learning could be. Teaching practice from my previous life as a teacher now seemed an easy undertaking compared to role-play in therapy training where we would alternate between taking on the role of therapist, child and observer. Becoming and remaining open to what was emerging from the learning, the interactions with the group, and in personal therapy proved challenging. What surfaced early on quickly debunked any preconceptions I had about the training: it was not going to be straightforward and it was definitely going to be very hard work. I discovered that I needed to look at, acknowledge and interrogate, my history, my ways of relating, my relationship to learning, my defences and coping strategies, and to give myself permission to feel vulnerable. What I learnt along the way was that this was an important and inevitable part of the training process but especially in the early weeks and months of the training, I often experienced it as a double bind: I wanted to be open to the process but that often rendered me vulnerable; and then I became anxious – at the root of it was the concern that I would be found wanting and deemed not fit to train as a therapist which, in turn, left me feeling more vulnerable. A diary extract from those early months depicts some of this struggle:

> *In my therapy session yesterday, I started to talk about feeling anxious all the time. I started to cry . . . and [my therapist] said she thought it was, once again, the "child within" needing to be seen and heard. I commented that the experience of training was bringing out a side of me I didn't know existed. [My therapist] said it was a question of coming in touch with 'little Elise'. Just writing this down makes me feel uncomfortable, that I am weak and feeble, not able to get on with things.*
>
> *(Personal journal, January 2003)*

Reading this back today reminds me so clearly of one of the early challenges I encountered: the belief developed over many years that in order to succeed, I just needed to be stronger, more focused, less anxious, not so emotional. But, in fact, the reverse became true: I needed to allow myself to open up to my vulnerabilities, to recognise that to become a therapist, perhaps especially a therapist working with children, I needed to give myself permission to access my inner child and to help her to heal. With the benefit not only of hindsight but also of the privilege of witnessing the training process of so many trainees in my role today as lecturer, I now understand my resistance more fully as well as the surprise and shock I felt that I could be so challenged by a process which I had initially thought would be a breeze rather than a storm.

The truth is I was naïve about what the process of training to be a therapist involved . . . and, after another session of personal therapy where all I could do was sit and cry, I initially wondered if I was disintegrating or falling apart, and questioned whether it meant I was not capable of being a therapist. I experienced shame and, as stated earlier, the fear of being found wanting, of not being up to the task, of being fundamentally flawed. But the feelings of being turned inside out, of being dismantled, of losing my previous professional identity before a new one was properly in sight . . . these were all part of the rich tapestry of "becoming" (Ayling et al., 2019) and a crucial part of ensuring that the trainee has engaged in personal development. I discovered I needed to embrace and trust in the process that I had embarked on.

Today in my role as a lecturer on the play therapy training, my aim is to support trainees to make sense of their training trajectory by contextualising and nor-malising their process of becoming. Of course, each process is individual and unique and does not change the complex nature of therapy training. It involves not only the academic rigour of a master's level training but also the crucial elements of personal development, such as personal therapy and experiential groups. The trainee grapples with lectures and assessments that throw new light on their his-tory, alongside immersing themselves in experiential learning with their training group. The trainee will experience periods of doubt, may feel shame and guilt, and will gradually become aware of parts of their core self that they were hitherto unfamiliar with (Luft, 1982). What happens next is crucial for the trainee's devel-opment. The trainee may be tempted to ignore what is emerging, to push it back down, to hide it away for to do otherwise may feel, temporarily, overwhelming and destabilising. However, for the process to be authentically meaningful and for the training to be grounding and effective, trainees must open themselves up to the process, to acknowledge and engage with the vulnerable parts of themselves. This helps the trainee to become aware of their own defences (Freud, 1993) and to ensure that they do not unconsciously block the client's process by being unaware of their internal proclivities. For instance, a trainee who may have difficulties with anger might unconsciously block the child's expression of anger if the trainee/ therapist has not worked through this emotion in their own therapy sessions and with their training group. The trainee also needs to find a way to articulate the shame and fear that may emerge. It is a process that renders the trainee vulner-able but it is in touching the core of one's own vulnerabilities that trainees and qualified therapists can sit alongside the vulnerable child as the process of play therapy unfolds.

## How did I arrive here? Motivations for training

Since becoming a lecturer on a play therapy training, I have become increasingly interested in the unconscious processes that often lead people into wanting to become therapists (Sussman, 1992). I was unaware of this at the start of my own training. The conscious impetus for my application for play therapy training was a clear wish to support children with emotional difficulties, borne out of many years of feeling frustrated with the limitations of a teacher's role in that regard. I recall arriving at a point where I felt I had done my time in education and needed a change. When research led me first to educational psychology, and then to play therapy, I was excited and believed that in play therapy I had found the perfect next step for me. I remember my play therapy interview clearly: I talked about my happy childhood, my years of working with children and young people, and my strong desire to help children and make a difference. "Perfect credentials" I thought. Today, after many years of interviewing play therapy candidates, I know that those who are offered a place on the training will often, just as I did, come to re-evaluate their reasons for wanting to train as play therapists. And many will find that they begin to understand their early childhood experiences in a different and more nuanced manner.

However, at the start of my training, I certainly did not fully understand or appreciate the way in which experiences beyond our conscious awareness can affect a person's development. The training brought into sharp focus the impact of early experiences on a child's emotional and psychological development, and attachment theory (Bowlby, 1969) provided me with a deeper understanding of the complex dance between infant and caregiver. I began to understand the implications of having been parented by my mother who developed severe postnatal depression after I was born, but initially I struggled to integrate this new knowledge.

According to Bowlby (1969), mental representations are formed through early interactions between the infant and their primary caregiver. These inner representations of the self and the other go on to shape the infant's expectations, perceptions and behaviours, providing the developing infant with a blueprint for approaching new situations. The infant develops internal working models of their "self", the "other" and the relationship between self and other (Bowlby, 1997). When a primary caregiver is not consistently responsive to the infant's needs, the infant will experience anxiety and distress, inhibiting them from developing a secure base. My family narrative was that I was a difficult baby who cried a lot and was hard to settle, which led to my mother being hospitalised for several weeks not long after I was born. For many years I believed my mother's hospital stay was my fault. But as I started to process my learning in personal therapy, I began to recognise how my mother's experience had shaped me in so many unconscious ways I had previously not been aware of.

As I processed this new knowledge and understanding, I began to look at my childhood experiences with a different lens and to appreciate the significant links between my history and why I was training to be a therapist. But re-evaluating my autobiography was challenging and, at the outset felt deeply unsettling and disloyal, especially to my mother. However, it also helped me to make sense of other experiences in my life and to construct a more coherent narrative of my childhood, recognising in the process that the wish to help children was much more complex and bound up in my history than I had previously been aware of.

> *This afternoon, [my therapist] suggested doing another "empty chair" exercise. I find these so challenging but I am allowing myself to engage much more honestly now. I decided to place my 6 year old self on the chair. Straightaway I felt I wanted to protect her, to make things better. I wanted to put my arms round her. . . . Sitting there, looking at 'young me', I really felt she needed help, and someone to understand her. . . . This training is making me appreciate the impact of an intervention like play therapy. I feel if there had been an adult in my childhood who could have given me the time to accept and understand myself, that I might have developed in a different way.*
>
> *(Personal journal, March 2003)*

I started school at almost 6 and, as an only child at the time, had rarely spent more than a couple of hours away from my mother. Separating from her was difficult for both of us. I developed psychosomatic symptoms, experiencing stomach cramps, nausea and disturbed sleep. All this took place in a country where in the 1960s, mental health awareness and provision for adults, much less children, were almost non-existent. Our family G.P. advised my mother to ignore my symptoms saying that I would soon get used to going to school. I learnt to adapt but experienced anxiety throughout my school years and often wondered why this was when I had friends and did reasonably well at school. Becoming a teacher was definitely an unconscious reparative drive.

My mother experienced recurring anxiety and depression throughout much of her adult life but a deep-seated mistrust of doctors meant she never sought active support for her condition until the final years of her life. Discovering the term "parentified child" (Boszormenyi-Nagy & Spark, 1984) helped me to understand the complex relationship I had with my mother in a more nuanced manner. The term is used to describe a subjective distortion in the parent-child role. This distortion of roles within the family system can result in the child attempting to fulfil the parental role, often at the expense of their own developmentally appropriate needs and pursuits. The parentified child becomes sensitive to their parent's moods, wishes and vulnerabilities, and will work hard to attune to the adult's needs (Chase cited in Castro et al., 2004). Training helped me develop awareness of how and why I responded in the way I did to myself, others and my environment. Insights emerged, sometimes slowly in a drip-drip effect in session after weekly session of personal therapy. At other times, insights dropped in like lightning bolts, a sudden flash of clarity lighting up my internal space with new understanding. Internal working models are believed to remain relatively stable over the life course. However, some researchers (Waters, Weinfield et al., 2000; Waters, Merrick et al., 2000) acknowledge that internal working models may be revised over time by new experiences. Therapy training became a transformational object (Bollas, 2012) for me and enabled me to work through the complex dynamics of my upbringing and adolescent years. Hooper (2007) hypothesised that an individual's attachment style and internal working models can become modified over time and this may explain how parentified children can experience different outcomes in adulthood. In my work today with trainees, I see this process of transformation in many of our students . . . those who slowly and determinedly accept the challenge to engage in a process of significant internal (and sometimes external) change. The trainees who embrace this personal work involved and went on to engage in deep psychotherapeutic relationships with the children they work with, helping them to process complex developmental issues such as abuse and trauma. Along with the capacity to process their therapeutic work using an integrated range of theories, such as psychoanalytic concepts from Infant Observation, attachment theory and others, these trainees can work effectively with complex cases. Other students who successfully complete the training may find their work takes them down a different path, perhaps one that focuses more on immediate and current issues. The work is still therapeutic and empowering for the child but the therapist may find themselves working at a more conscious level with the child and in a more therapist-led manner. Settings and organisational requirements also play a part in the type of work therapists find themselves engaged in post-qualification. However, much also seems to depend on the extent to which the trainee is willing to open themselves up to personal development and change.

## Transitions: trainee to newly hatched therapist

Whilst training was demanding, I found the transition to post-qualification practice created new challenges, on both personal and professional levels. The process of engaging in therapy and personal development brought certain aspects of my life before training into sharp focus. I became much more aware of the internal constraints I had experienced from living in a tiny country that at the time was largely homogenous in both ethnicity and culture. Society at all levels was strongly influenced by a conservative approach to religion. In my therapy, I explored my experience of growing up in such a traditional environment where societal roles were determined by gender, where religious mores were a mother who was not Maltese and therefore not part of the dominant culture. I was able to put words to the experience growing up always feeling a little bit different, something of an outsider, not quite belonging. That and my insecurities meant I often hung back, remained silent and tried to merge into the background. Some of my work in therapy focused on finding my voice. An extract from a poem I wrote during my training articulates something of this process:

*. . . A voice deep within, a strength*
*That accepts, validates and empowers . . .*
*It is ok to speak*
*I have a voice*
*And a life within*

*I am allowed*
*To have my perspective*
*My experience . . .*
*No one can take that away*
*No one can deny me it.*
*It is ok to speak*
*My witness has given me a voice*
*Has given me the power*
*To be heard*
*To be able to say 'No'*
*And face the consequences*
*To say 'Yes'*
*And stay with the demands . . .*

*I want to be true to myself . . .*
*I may not conform*
*To others' expectations of me*
*And that is ok.*
                    *(Personal journal, June 2003)*

As the time approached when I would have to start making plans to return home to Malta, I began to realise I had some difficult choices to make. The room with the sink beckoned but I became increasingly uncertain about whether I wanted to return to my "old life". I was aware that it would be very easy, in some ways, just to slip back and pick up where I had left off. I would be the only play therapist on the island, I could develop my practice exactly as I wanted to and I could make a real difference. And yet on a personal level, I knew it would be infinitely harder: the thought of returning to my home country started to feel repressive, constricting and suffocating. I began to grapple with the thoughts about whether I was prepared to remain true to what I had discovered about myself during my training and personal therapy; whether I was prepared to make choices that might confuse, disappoint and hurt those closest to me because the alternative would be a betrayal of what I now knew I needed to live a healthy and authentic life. One of my training peers had shared a poem with us towards the end of our training and it captured something of my difficult dilemma:

> It doesn't interest me if the story you're telling me is true.
> I want to know if you can disappoint another – to be true to yourself.
> If you can bear the accusation of betrayal and not betray your own soul.
> (Oriah Mountain Dreamer, 2000)

I decided to stay in the United Kingdom.

And yet, perhaps unsurprisingly, that decision came at a cost. I found myself alone in a still "new" country and in anonymous London. It was great in the heady days of training when there was always a group of peers to return to and connect with, but much harder when I found myself living alone and trying to develop a new career without any previous work places or connections to fall back on. But I was determined to stay, and now could . . . following a referendum, Malta became a member of the EU whilst I was in training, which meant I could reside as an EU citizen. And, in a quirky irony, during the course of writing this chapter, I have had to apply for "settled status": the result of another referendum, this time the United Kingdom voting to leave the EU.

In developing my post-qualification experience, I encountered the common challenge of being qualified and yet realising there was a great deal I still did not know (Skovholt & Rønnestad, 2003). The concept of conscious incompetence (Clarkson & Gilbert, 1988) is relevant here and useful in the context of beginning therapy practice. As I attended interviews and, later, began work as a qualified play therapist, I found myself feeling challenged by the awareness of still having a lot to learn and yet feeling pressure, both internal and external, that I was now qualified and therefore "should be" competent. It was at this time that I began to grapple with feelings of doubt which were different to those encountered during training. Experiencing self-doubt on the training felt acceptable: there was a training group and we were all learning together. Even though there were times when I compared myself unfavourably to others, I could conceptualise it as part of the training process, and part of my work in supervision whilst training was exploring the emerging proclivities and new insights. But for a while after qualifying, until I began to articulate the doubt and feelings of incompetence (Cuschieri, 2016) in personal therapy and in supervision, I judged myself harshly, deciding I was failing in my practice, that I should not be experiencing doubt in myself and my practice because I was now qualified and needed to demonstrate professional competence and confidence.

Chase (Chase cited in Castro et al., 2004) argues that parentified children will frequently experience anxiety as adults and often worry about being unable to meet the demands and expectations that they place on themselves. As I began practising, I experienced this more profoundly than I ever had as a teacher. The self-doubt grew inside me as did the feeling that I was not worthy to do this type of delicate emotional work. Clance and Imes (1978) describe this type of self-doubt as "the impostor phenomenon" and postulate that impostors harbour feelings of incompetence and fear that they will fail to live up to the expectations of themselves and of others (Clance, 1985). The loneliness of feeling that I was the only one struggling with these powerful feelings was, at times, depleting and isolating. However, over the years, from conversations with other play therapists, students and therapists from other disciplines, I now realise that this is not as uncommon or unique as I once thought it to be. Committing my thoughts about self-doubt to paper (Cuschieri, 2016) was a challenging but personally valuable experience. I could not look at my chapter for several months (maybe years even . . .) after its publication, but several people from a range of backgrounds in therapeutic practice contacted me to say that they identified with some of the feelings I had attempted to articulate. And within our training programme, discussions opened up with students about some of the challenges students and qualified therapists experience. I found this stimulating and fulfilling, and it made committing my vulnerabilities to a published document feel like a worthwhile risk.

Skovholt and Rønnestad (2003) discuss the lack of professional confidence in novice therapists. They go on to suggest that the confidence more experienced practitioners have serves to buffer anxiety when difficulties are encountered. I certainly recognise this when I first started practising and recall a particular instance a few months into my first job as a play therapist when a child suddenly refused to come to the playroom with me. I had been working with George[1] for a few weeks. He was an anxious and reserved child who had been referred for play therapy due to witnessing domestic abuse. I felt we were developing a trusting relationship but on this occasion, when I went to collect him from a waiting area crowded with people, he turned away from me and clutched his mother tightly. She told me he did not want to have his session today but that she had encouraged him to come to the centre. As she spoke, I felt as though all eyes in the waiting area were suddenly focused on me. I felt self-conscious and immediately incompetent: how could I expect to be a play therapist if a child would not even come to the playroom with me? I experienced my body responding to the rising anxiety: my knee started to tremble, my heart raced and I became very flushed. In that moment, I could not enter into George's world and empathise with the difficulties he was facing because what was happening within me was distracting. Skovholt and Rønnestad (2003) posit that self-consciousness, which causes novice therapists to over-focus on themselves, makes it more difficult to attend to, and manage, the complex tasks of the therapeutic process. The situation with George was over in a matter of minutes. I invited George and his mother to a quieter, more private area, and found out that due to a mistake by the allocated social worker, George's father, who was the alleged perpetrator of the domestic abuse, had found out where they were living. George did not want to leave his mother because he was fearful. We talked for a few minutes and, in that time, I was able to ground myself sufficiently to attend to what George needed, which was to be with his mother that day.

But, as a general experience in the early months and years of post-qualification practice, I know I felt challenged on a regular basis by feelings of self-consciousness and incompetence, as well as an increasing awareness of the phenomenon of ambiguity. As I began my play therapy practice, I realised that what I had learnt in my training could not always be applied in a straightforward and logical manner to practice. I questioned what my role as a play therapist should look like in practice and the oft-quoted maxim in therapy trainings "trust the process" seemed singularly unhelpful in those early weeks and months. Starting to process referrals myself and having to liaise with other professionals as well as the families seeking support proved complex; and the concept I had built up in training that the referral and therapeutic processes were linear had to be revised. I became much more sensitive to the complexity of human systems, both client groups and professional organisations, but a lack of confidence as a novice therapist meant I was prone to viewing situations as being definite and unambiguous. In practice, I had to develop a capacity for tolerating ambiguity and to learn to be very patient. Today I recognise that so much of the work in the field of psychotherapy is coloured by ambiguity because the focus is on the emotional world of humans, and this seems especially true for therapists working with children where metaphor and symbolism in play often mean we do not always understand straightaway what is being communicated. I often found myself wondering whether what I was doing was "real therapy" or whether I was "just" playing with a child. I frequently felt fraudulent and sometimes guilty. Again, Skovholt and Rønnestad (1997) helpfully expand on their research with beginning therapists which found that at the affective level, the therapist who is not yet familiar with their new professional role feels both enthusiasm and insecurity. They (2003: 46) note that "Expertise within the web of ambiguity takes years to master". This certainly resonates with my experience then and I find the following a useful reminder when working with students today:

> Creating a practitionerself, a term similar to that of Ellwein, Grace, and Comfort (1990), involves vigorous internal construction work, as well as the external effort of trying on new clothes and new ways of being in the world. Like an adolescent, the fragile and incomplete practitionerself shifts through a series of moods: enthusiasm, insecurity, elation, fear, relief, frustration, delight, despair, pride, and shame. The novice self is fragile and, therefore, highly reactive to negative feedback. Metaphorically expressed, there is not much muscle, and the immunology system is stressed.
>
> (Skovholt & Rønnestad, 2003: 50)

But in starting to articulate feelings of doubt and incompetence, and a sense of being an imposter (Clance & Imes, 1978), I was better able to understand the challenges of early post-qualifying practice and to recognise the trajectory from unconscious incompetence through to conscious incompetence, conscious competence and, somewhere along the line unconscious competence (Clarkson &

Gilbert, 1988). Jung's concept of the wounded healer (Sedgwick, 2016; Cvetovac & Adame, 2017) was also helpful in beginning to understand the relationship between my own wounds and my identity as a developing therapist.

## Some concluding thoughts about the process of "becoming"

Over the years, since developing my post-qualifying play therapy practice and then beginning work as a lecturer on a master's play therapy training programme, I have reflected a great deal on my process and developmental trajectory, as well as that of the trainees I work with. The following has helped me to think about key processes and when teaching today, I hold in mind what I have notionally termed the 3 A's, namely: **Awareness, Acceptance and Authenticity**. I should acknowledge that I come from a background of teaching in both primary and secondary education, where in the latter role, I taught English. I have always enjoyed playing around with sounds and words so I could not allow the opportunity to "alliterate" pass me by. Nevertheless, I believe that these three words elucidate an important developmental trajectory for the trainee and novice therapist, which I see as being both linear and circular.

At the start of training, the learning curve is often fairly straight and very steep but, as the trainee grows and develops, the process becomes more of a circular progression as new knowledge comes into awareness and the trainee/novice therapist seeks to understand, accept and integrate it so as to respond authentically both to their self and to the child/family they are working with.

The first crucial step in this process is developing **awareness**. This happens in a myriad of ways during training, from lectures and seminars, to experiential groups, play therapy placement practice and personal therapy. In all these situations, students are encouraged to develop their awareness on many levels – cognitively not only through their reading and participation in lectures but also emotionally, psychologically and, critically I believe, of their body: to become aware of the subtle and imperceptible messages that they receive from their bodies during the course of training, and to be curious about these often fleeting messages – something is talked about, shared and discussed, and there may be an unconscious shutting off, turning away, closing down, as psychological defences come into play. For genuine awareness to develop, it is crucial for the trainee to be curious about what is behind such responses, what is being communicated on an unconscious level and what can be learnt from it. By attuning to their bodies, and becoming aware of all the clues, communications and messages that their bodies hold when interacting with others, trainees can deepen awareness and understanding of themselves.

Personal therapy also plays a valuable and vital role in this process. In relationship with their therapist, the trainee has the opportunity to develop their reflective capacity. As the therapeutic relationship grows, and trust develops between trainee and therapist, the trainee has the time and space to cultivate a deeper understanding of their self in relation to their inner world and to others. As awareness develops, and new insights emerge, the trainee has the opportunity to start to explore those vulnerabilities that may be impeding their capacity to relate in an open and congruent manner with the other. This developmental process is crucial for the trainee in creating new ways to understand themselves first and, later, the children they work with: to engage their whole person in interacting with the child and thus being open to whatever the child is communicating – verbally, non-verbally and through their play.

With awareness comes the critical need for **acceptance**. First of all, acceptance of self: the need for the trainee to accept their self wholly and totally so as to be able to genuinely accept the other. The Rogerian concept of unconditional positive regard (Rogers, 1951) is complex and challenging, perhaps the most demanding of the "core conditions". For those trainees and therapists who are familiar with a critical inner voice, the challenge can be even greater: how does one offer genuine unconditional positive regard to the child when one's own internal dialogue is not unconditional? Over the years, from my own experiences, I have come to realise that this is a pivotal element in many trainees' and new therapists' developmental trajectory. Becoming more accepting and compassionate with oneself is a crucial step, which can only be fully realised and experienced between therapist and child if therapists strive to unconditionally accept, and have unconditional positive regard towards themselves. This is an easily stated but, often, challenging concept.

With awareness and acceptance of self, then there is the opportunity to develop **authenticity** in relationships. For trainees, the task is often to dig deep, to develop in self-knowledge, understanding and insight. For it is in committing to this deep personal development that the trainee is able to strive towards genuine and congruent relations so that the relationship they develop in their practice with the child is authentic, alive and real, moment by moment.

Learning about the concept of the "false self" (Winnicott, 2018) helped me to further understand the importance of authenticity in relation to my own development as an infant and child. The false self develops as the infant learns that to be accepted and loved by the other, they need to respond, behave and react in certain ways. The child consciously or unconsciously hides their true feelings behind the false self and may become compliant in order to be loved and accepted. As discussed earlier, the personal therapy component in my training and beyond supported me in becoming aware of my experiences as an infant, child and adolescent. I was able to acknowledge and accept the attachment strategies (Bowlby, 2005) I had developed unconsciously as an infant and had brought with me into adulthood. This insight enabled me to work on healing the hurt child within me and to slowly allow my authentic self to emerge. Bonovitz (2009) talks about how the therapist's own childhood experiences may be brought to the surface when working with children. He also discusses how these experiences can produce new meaning for the therapist in the intersubjective context of therapeutic work with a child. This was a helpful perspective in my development and alerted me in particular to those children whom I recognised as having similar (but crucially not "the same") histories as my own and who had adapted and adjusted to their environment by developing similar attachment strategies. Such children have always proved to be invaluable unconscious teachers and I am indebted to them.

In bringing this chapter to its conclusion, I am reminded again of the immense privilege I feel at being able to work with both children and their families in a therapeutic process and with trainees through their individual journeys of "becoming". Both require delicate, sensitive and patient work, taking one small step after another, not rushing ahead, not making assumptions, trusting in the human capacity to grow and develop . . . joining in the process of the other and in doing so, experiencing the phenomenon so fittingly expressed by Jung (Jung et al., 2001) that "The meeting of two personalities is like the contact of two chemical substances: if there is any reaction, both are transformed". This is certainly my experience and I close by acknowledging all the children and families I have worked with over the years, and the trainees who have undertaken play therapy training – thank you for teaching me so much.

## Note

1 Pseudonym.

## References

Axline, V. M. (1989) *Play Therapy*. Edinburgh and New York: Churchill Livingstone.

Axline, V. M. (1990) *Dibs: In Search of Self*. London: Penguin.

Ayling, P., Armstrong, H. & Gordon Clark, L. (2019) *Becoming and Being a Play Therapist*. London: Routledge.

Bollas, C. (2012) *The Christopher Bollas Reader*. London: Routledge.

Bonovitz, C. (2009). Countertransference in Child Psychoanalytic Psychotherapy: The Emergence of the Analyst's Childhood. *Psychoanalytic Psychology*, 26(3), pp. 235–245.

Boszormenyi-Nagy, I. & Spark, G. M. (1984) *Invisible Loyalties: Reciprocity in Intergenerational Family Therapy*. New York: Brunner/Mazel.

Bowlby, J. (1969) *Attachment and Loss*. New York: Basic Books.

Bowlby, J. (1997) *Attachment and Loss. Vol. 1*. London: Pimlico.

Bowlby, J. (2005) *A Secure Base: Clinical Applications of Attachment Theory*. London: Routledge (Routledge classics).

Castro, D. M., Jones, R. A. & Mirsalimi, H. (2004) Parentification and the Impostor Phenomenon: An Empirical Investigation. *The American Journal of Family Therapy*, 32(3), pp. 205–216. DOI: 10.1080/01926180490425676.

Clance, P. R. (1985) *Imposter Phenomenon*. Atlanta, GA: Peachtree.

Clance, P. R. & Imes, S. A. (1978) The Imposter Phenomenon in High Achieving Women: Dynamics and Therapeutic Intervention. *Psychotherapy: Theory, Research & Practice*, 15(3), pp. 241–247. https://doi.org/10.1037/h0086006.

Clarkson, P. & Gilbert, M. (1988) The Training of Counsellors and Supervisors. In: Dryden, W. & Thorne, B. (eds.) *Training and Supervision for Counselling in Action*. London: Sage.

Cuschieri, E. (2016) Can I Really Do This? An Exploration Into Therapist Self-Doubt. In Le Vay, D. & Cuschieri, E. (eds.) *Challenges in the Theory and Practice of Play Therapy*. London: Routledge.

Cvetovac, M. E. & Adame, A. L. (2017) The Wounded Therapist: Understanding the Relationship Between Personal Suffering and Clinical Practice. *The Humanistic Psychologist*, 45(4), 348–366. https://doi.org/10.1037/hum0000071.

Freud, A. (1993) *The Ego and the Mechanisms of Defence* (Rev. ed.). London: Karnac Books and the Institute of Psycho-Analysis.

Hooper, L. (2007) The Application of Attachment Theory and Family Systems Theory to the Phenomenon of Parentification. *The Family Journal*, 15(3), pp. 217–223. DOI: 10.1177/1066480707301290.

Jung, C. G., Dell, W. S. & Baynes, C. F. (2001) *Modern Man in Search of a Soul*. London: Routledge (Routledge classics).

Luft, J. (1982) *The Johari Window: A Graphic Model of Awareness in Interpersonal Relations*. Available at: www.convivendo.net/wp-content/uploads/2009/05/johari-window-articolo-originale.pdf (Accessed: 9 August 2021).

Oriah Mountain Dreamer. (2000) *The Invitation*. San Francisco: Harper.

Rogers, C. (1951) *Client Centred Therapy: Its Current Practice, Implications and Theory* Reprint. London: Little, Brown Book Group, 1995.

Sedgwick, D. (2016) *The Wounded Healer: Countertransference from a Jungian Perspective* (2nd ed.). London: Taylor and Francis (Routledge Mental Health Classic Editions). Available at: http://public.ebookcentral.proquest.com.roe.idm.oclc.org/choice/public-fullrecord.aspx?p=4560428 (Accessed: 21 November 2021).

Skovholt, T. M. & Rønnestad, M. H. (1997) *The Evolving Professional Self: Stages and Themes in Therapist and Counselor Development*. Chichester: Wiley.

Skovholt, T. M. & Rønnestad, M. H. (2003) Struggles of the Novice Counselor and Therapist. *Journal of Career Development*, 30(1), pp. 45–58.

Sussman, M. B. (1992) *A Curious Calling: Unconscious Motivations for Practicing Psychotherapy*. Landham, MD: Jason Aronson.

Waters, E., Merrick, S., Treboux, D., Crowell, J. & Albersheim, L. (2000) Attachment Security in Infancy and Early Adulthood: A Twenty-Year Longitudinal Study. *Child Development*, 71(3), pp. 684–689.

Waters, E., Weinfield, N. S. & Hamilton, C. E. (2000) The Stability of Attachment Security from Infancy to Adolescence and Early Adulthood: General Discussion. *Child Development*, 71(3), 703–706. https://doi.org/10.1111/1467-8624.00179.

Wikipedia Contributors. (2019) *Malta*. Wikipedia. Available at: https://en.wikipedia.org/wiki/Malta (Accessed: 9 July 2021).

Winnicott, D. W. (2018) *The Maturational Processes and the Facilitating Environment: Studies in the Theory of Emotional Development*. Abingdon, Oxon: Routledge. Available at: https://ebookcentral.proquest.com/lib/roehampton-ebooks (Accessed: 20 August 2021).

# Chapter 3

# The stories we tell about ourselves

*Lauren Shaw*

For every therapist, the personal process of training and therapeutic practice is unique. We all come to the decision to train in the helping professions for myriad reasons and, also, we each bring our past experiences, thoughts, behaviours, feelings and personal narratives. Virginia Satir (1987: 17) suggests that

> [T]herapy is a deeply intimate and vulnerable experience, requiring sensitivity to one's own state of being as well as to that of the other. It is the meeting of the deepest self of the therapist with the deepest self of the patient or client.

It is therefore self-evident that the "personhood" or "self" of the therapist is present, regardless of therapeutic approach or tools utilised (Satir, 1987). So what, then, of those physicians who bring with them their own struggles or "wounds"? How does this impact on their professional identity and practice? The archetype of the "wounded healer" has been at the forefront of my mind when thinking about my personal process, from child client to adult practitioner. My own "woundedness" as a survivor of intrafamilial childhood sexual abuse (CSA) has had far-reaching impacts. As a construct, the wounded healer has been afforded little academic attention and is often misunderstood or romanticised (Zerubavel & O'Dougherty Wright, 2012). However, through personal experience and extensive documentation, it is evident that, for many therapists, a history of pain or suffering is often a precursor to arriving at their profession of choice (Barnett, 2007; Farber et al., 2005; Zerubavel & O'Dougherty Wright, 2012). My choice to become a play therapist was threefold. Crucially, my belief in the efficacy of play therapy, following my own first-hand and transformative childhood experience of the process; secondly, my want to help and support children and families to navigate their way through their own personal struggles; thirdly, my desire to give children what I craved and needed as a child: the experience of an adult who listens, understands and gives a voice to help tell one's stories and shape one's future. For me, however, the process of becoming the therapist I am today has not followed a straight trajectory – child client, trainee, therapist. It has instead been a journey of self-exploration, self-discovery and learning that will continue throughout, not only my career, but the rest of my life.

DOI: 10.4324/9781003017271-3

## *"O Mighty One"*

As a play therapy practitioner, it would be remiss of me if I did not give attention to where my passion and belief in the practice began. This is because play therapy not only enabled me to explore my difficult life experiences during childhood, but it has also given me unique insight into the play therapy process as an adult practitioner, informing the way in which I practice and relate to children and families.

Eighteen years ago, I stepped through the door of a woman who was to ignite my fascination with the world of play therapy and who would change my world irrevocably. She was playful, she did not just speak to my parents *but to me too*, looking me in the eye, asking me how I felt and for my perspective on what had brought me to her. She spoke in an inclusive and kind way. She did not shy away, or recoil, when discussing the years of sexual abuse perpetrated by my grandfather towards me and several members of my family. Unlike all other adults around me, she was not scared to talk about it openly, pulling it up by its roots and removing its power. I could not put my finger on exactly why, but I felt "normal" in her presence. I was not the sexually abused nine-year-old girl; I was just me, a child stood in a room full of toys that would become the canvas on which to tell my story. I spent the next four years intermittently accessing her service. It was a permissive space without pressure, allowing exploration of my experiences. It was *my* time and space to explore what *I* wanted, in the *way* I wanted, in the presence of my play therapist, who I idolised and trusted to help me move on; the sessions acted as a vehicle for me to tolerably continue my life.

Narrative and the use of stories were something that my therapist emphasised. She was a story maker with a fantastic imagination and a flare for characterisation. For children who have experienced sexual abuse, the play therapy process can be tempestuous. A narrative approach to therapy with abused children is often utilised; this is based on narrative therapy and social construction theory which Cattanach (2008: 5) describes as the "development of identity based on the stories we tell about ourselves and the stories others . . . tell about us". Sexually abused children often have dominant stories imposed upon them by the perpetrators of the abuse, these being subsequently reinforced by societal reactions upon disclosure (Cattanach, 2008). These stories are often disorganised and, in my experience, can leave the child with feelings of responsibility and shame. My exploration of these narratives, through my own symbolic role-plays allowed me a safe distance at which to process my experiences. I slipped in and out of different characters, trying them on like one would a pair of shoes. Some felt comfortable and almost familiar, whilst others hurt and rubbed and were hard to bear. I would sometimes become overwhelmed, as my role-plays began to feel too real, and memories flooded my mind and senses. My play therapist, who was attuned to my states and internal world, would gently guide me back to reality and make me feel safe again. Although this was not always an easy process, we were able to explore alternative narratives and solutions and expand themes in an effort to help make sense of my abusive experiences. This allowed me to find ways of functioning that did not re-process previous patterns of negative relationships and behaviours (Cattanach, 2008; Gil, 1991; Landreth, 2012). The narrative that I created for myself, with her gentle guidance and support, was one of a strong and empowered young woman who would not be defined by her traumatic experiences.

I was also learning about myself in relation to my therapist (Axline, 1969; Cattanach, 2008). In my childhood diary, I referred to her as *"O Mighty One"*. On reflection, the reason for this is that she not only had the ability to create feelings of safety and permissiveness within the playroom, but also, through disclosure of her own experience of childhood sexual abuse (CSA), she made me recognise I was not alone. In Feminist Therapy (Gefter et al., 2013) and Group Therapy (Yalom, 1985), sharing of abusive experiences is pivotal in sexual abuse survivor's recovery process. My play therapist's disclosure of abuse was not discussed explicitly; it was a part of her "being", reflected in the inclusive and informed language that she used: "us", "we", "it makes you feel . . .", "I felt . . .". I was not ashamed to tell her my story because, in a way, it was our story, and that of all others who have survived this injustice. I drew extreme strength and comfort from this. She appeared to understand my pain deeply because, as Goethe wrote ". . . our own suffering prepares us to appreciate the suffering of others" (Zerubavel & O'Dougherty Wright, 2012: 482). Her self-disclosure and her defiance against perpetrators having power over those they target was an extremely healing part of my time within play therapy. It gave me hope that I would one day heal and "recover" from the immense pain and hurt that I felt and that I too would be as resilient and powerful as her. It was not just the words that she spoke that exuded strength and hope of recovery, but it was also through her physical presence. There was something solid about her, an intangible quality that told me everything was going to be alright. In my other relationships and conversations with adults who were aware of my past experiences, it was apparent that the fact I had been sexually abused made them uncomfortable. This was either because of the emotions and memories it triggered in them or because they did not know the words that would make everything "okay" again. This sense of discomfort was often not portrayed by what they said but, instead, through their body language and physical presence. They would shrink into themselves or they would find it hard to be in close proximity to me, turning their bodies and faces away and minimising eye contact. This heightened the feeling of "difference" that I already felt. I had become very much attuned to this shift in physical presence within my personal relationships and I was both delighted and reassured when my play therapist was unchanged by my disclosures. She remained solid, present, alert and comfortable throughout our time together.

Self-disclosure of abuse from a play therapist to their client is not common practice; a degree of anonymity is seen as customary; it is thought by some that therapist self-disclosure is a tool that meets the needs of the therapist rather than those of the child, placing feelings of responsibility onto the child, thus shifting the power balance within the therapeutic relationship (Landreth, 2012). This is not something I ever questioned or explored until I entered into my own play therapy training.

When I decided it was time for my therapy to end, I truly believed that my journey of recovery was over. I was now a teenager and I wanted to completely rid myself of the "otherness" that I had felt in my pre-teen years and feel located within the social group of which I was part, a group that seemed enticingly carefree and unconcerned with "darker matters". I felt confident to step away from therapy and the therapeutic relationship because I knew that, if I wished, I could return. My therapist conveyed, through her use of language, that our ending was open-ended and that there was no finite end to the relationship we had formed. I trusted my play therapist to hold my story and memories as I embarked on this new stage in my life, although I still hosted my "demons". They were repressed and unspoken, but part of my being (Braham, 1995). Play therapy and the traumatic memories that accompanied it would fall into the shadows for many years until I was once again ready to return to them. Only then would I realise that "recovery is not necessarily linear or, when achieved, permanent, contributing to the complexity of assessing a wounded healers' recovery status" (Zerubavel & O'Dougherty Wright, 2012: 485).

## Unearthing old wounds

Creating a personal narrative is crucial: we make sense of our lives through the stories we create (McAdams, 2006). From ceasing play therapy (13 years old) to beginning my MA Play Therapy training (25 years old), my personal narrative was fixed: I had dealt with my past trauma, had a reasonable recollection of events, knew the thoughts, feelings and impact that learning about my sexually abusive experiences and my subsequent therapy had on my parents. I had been able to "move on", leaving the past firmly behind. I felt confident that my own wounds would allow me insight and could enable me to support others with minimal negative emotional impact. This was, however, a narrative that would be reshaped, explored, challenged and changed during my training.

I was prepared for the Play Therapy Masters Level Training Programme to be a rigorous pursuit. I had prepared myself by researching the programme and felt ready for the academic demands of the course. I felt I possessed some of the personal qualities desirous in a play therapy candidate: "emotional literacy, robustness and an ability to be self-reflective" (Gordon Clark, 2019: 12). This initial certainty was, in hindsight, naïve as I had underestimated the impact that engaging in therapeutic work with clients, in a relational context, would have. When discussing the training process, Aponte and Winter (1987: 94) proffered that "there are aspects of the person of the therapist that are specifically, and often only, revealed to the clinician through [their] conduct of therapy". This was certainly true for me. I noticed that thoughts and feelings, particularly those pertaining to the sexual abuse suffered in my childhood and my own play therapy process, began to come to the fore. This was initially daunting; I knew that I would need to address these feelings if I was to effectively support others and was alarmed that my personal narrative appeared less faithful than I had believed. Had I resolved my past traumas? Did I have the ability to acknowledge my own internal damaged child?

Braham (1995: 37) posits that "we see the past . . . in something of the same way we see a Henry Moore sculpture. The 'holes' define the 'shape'. What is left repressed, or what cannot be uttered, is often as significant to the whole shape of the life as what is said". I had, perhaps, not acknowledged some experiences as part of my whole being and found addressing these within the context of the course too threatening. During the first year of training, it felt riskier to disclose my own woundedness to my cohort and tutors, as I feared judgement towards my ability to support the children and families I was working with and my ability to resolve my own wounds and their impact (Zerubavel & O'Dougherty Wright, 2012). I was also preoccupied, during the initial sessions with children, with the need to "get it right"; therapeutic responses, body language, vocal inflections, active listening and observing. It was only within the safe confines of personal therapy sessions that I began to explore my emerging feelings and what this might mean for my practice and therapeutic process. It was not until the second year of training that I would feel comfortable enough in my abilities as a play therapist and in my own personal strength to begin to fully explore my personal process and to scrutinise my inner world, sifting the impact of my clients from the background noise of my own personal domain (Lanyado, 2004).

As our client base became more complex during our second-year placement, and lectures and theoretical learning began to focus on some of the more vulnerable populations within our client demographic, I became increasingly frustrated with the negative prognosis regarding the future for these individuals. I was particularly interested in the group in which I was located: those who had suffered childhood sexual abuse. It appeared that most researchers aimed to give a generalised picture of the long-term effects following disclosure, often focusing on the most common and severe effects: post-traumatic stress disorder (PTSD), depression, suicide, sexualised behaviours and re-victimisation (Beitchman et al., 1992; Briere & Elliott, 1994; Putnam, 2003). My fellow trainees also regularly voiced surprise and delight when hearing of a child who had experienced CSA and had gone on to live a happy and "normal" life. I found that much of the research and perceived prognosis of my friends and fellow practitioners did not represent my experiences, due to the paucity of voices and insights of the survivors themselves. This lack of understanding regarding the subtleties the experiences of survivors and the shortage of survivors' voices within research left me feeling "other than". I wrestled with the thought, "am I more damaged than I think?" I soon realised that, although I had my demons and triggers just like everyone else, I was not "damaged" and nor were other CSA survivors that I knew who had received adequate support. My concerns morphed into feelings of anger and injustice. I wanted to change and challenge these preconceptions, not just for myself, but for all negatively impacted by this mystifying omission. I also wanted people (particularly trainee practitioners) to recognise play therapy's positive effect on children's future trajectories.

I knew that I wanted to use my own experiences of intrafamilial CSA and reflections on my childhood play therapy sessions to inform my dissertation. I was in a quandary as to how I would tackle such a large and personal topic. My preliminary research indicated that first-person narrative research on CSA is limited; autoethnographic and feminist approaches are forerunners in changing this within professional literature by emphasising the voice of the survivor (Christensen, 2011; Metta, 2010; Gefter et al., 2013; Scott, 2001). I therefore felt compelled to use autoethnography as my approach.

I chose to title my autoethnographic paper, *"The Ripple Effect of Disclosure: An Insight into the 'Lived Experience' Following Disclosure of Intrafamilial Childhood Sexual Abuse and Reflections on the Role of Play Therapy in Such Circumstances"*. This was supported by three sub-questions that provided structure and focus to my research: (1) *What are the positive and negative impacts of play therapy for those effected by intrafamilial CSA? (2) How is loss, in any form, experienced following disclosure of intrafamilial CSA? (3) What impact does intrafamilial CSA have on the survivor's sense of self and how does the sense of self shift over time?*

> Auto-ethnography is an approach to research and writing that seeks to describe and systemically analyse (*graphy*) personal experience (*auto*) in order to understand cultural experience (*ethno*) (Ellis et al., 2011; Holman-Jones, 2005). This approach challenges canonical ways of doing research and representing others (Spry, 2001) and treats research as political, socially-just and socially-conscious act (Adams & Holman Jones, 2008). A researcher uses tenets of *autobiography* and *ethnography* to *do* and *write* auto-ethnography Thus, as a method, auto-ethnography is both process and product.
>
> (Ellis et al., 2011)

For me, the autoethnographic *process* that led to the finished *product* was both life-changing and deeply emotional. What started out as a politically and socially just act that aimed to give people first-hand insight into the lived experience following disclosure of intra-familial CSA, evolved at my fingertips and became something much bigger. It not only shone a light onto the nuances of experience and helped to demonstrate that, with the right therapeutic support, children can begin to heal after suffering sexual abuse, but it also enabled me to gain a deeper understanding of myself (past and present), those closest to me and the kind of therapist I wanted to become.

## The wounded healer: reconnecting with the past

At the commencement of my autoethnographic project, I believed that I had a reasonable recollection of events from my past. This was not the case. My lack of clarity brought with it a sense of powerlessness. It also made me doubt my capacity to write an autoethnographic paper that was true and faithful to my experiences. I knew that the autoethnographic process relied on taking data such as field notes, interviews, artefacts, and then describing them "using facets of storytelling (e.g. character and plot development), showing and telling, and alterations of authorial voice" (Ellis et al., 2011). I had a wealth of historical artefacts; these included family photos, letters between myself and my grandparents, post-disclosure, diaries, drawings and a DVD copy of my police interview from 2000. My parents and childhood play therapist had also consented to partake in Reflexive-Dyadic interviews. My difficulty was, however, in my ability to capture the voices and experiences of my multiple "selves" that existed in different times and contexts (Christensen, 2011): researcher-self, remembering-self, past-self.

On leaving play therapy, I had put everything into a physical box and had learnt to disassociate. I was now struggling to reconnect to my past self, who I will refer to as "Little Lauren". Dissociation is an adaptive response that Van der Kolk (2014: 180) describes as 'creating a dual memory system': the traumatic memories do not integrate with the continuous flow of autobiographical memory. As a teenager I had felt that my personal narrative fell outside the "norm" and that it would be misunderstood, resulting in judgement. To avoid rejection, my story became a rote narrative of a strong, powerful and unaffected individual (Christensen, 2011; Van der Kolk, 2014). I now had a deep want and need to connect to Little Lauren. I knew that it was not just an integral part of my research project but also my growth as a therapist: as Sue Jennings (1993:147) proffers, "if we choose to work with damaged children then we must be prepared to acknowledge our own internal damaged child".

I believed that the turning point in my "remembering" would be my interview with my childhood play therapist. It was hoped that her recollection of my time within play therapy would be my point of connection. I viewed her as "keeper of my memories and experiences"; surely our sessions were as precious to her as they were to me? However, our discussion revealed that she remembered very little. In that moment, the therapeutic illusion was broken. My respect for her was not diminished; instead, my perception was altered. I was able to see her as human and fallible, as opposed to my childhood view of her as almost "superhuman". There was no anger on my part; I still felt that she had kept Little Lauren safe so that she could shape her life. Until the interview, my therapist remained, in my mind, a figure of strength and protector of children, during a time when I could not connect to my traumatic past.

I explored her "forgetting" in the form of a poem.

### "So I haven't enlightened you"

Memories fade into dust,
I thought they were ones that I could trust.
Keeper of secrets, keeper of past,
Just like mine, they didn't last.

I see the anguish in your face,
Desperately searching for any trace.
What does this mean for the children of play,
That come to you searching on a later day?

I see you now, human and fallible,
The hero I idolised, a woman so magical.
Sits before me, still a figure of hope,
If you were unrecognisable, I just couldn't cope.

But your image has changed,
There is just something different.
I can't put my finger on it,
But it's not insignificant.

It is me! I have changed.
Now we sit here as peers,
But you were the woman
Who took all my fears.

(a poem of lost memories)

(Written, May 2017)

My play therapist commented during interview, "*so I haven't enlightened you*", sensing my disappointment. Although disappointed that this interview did not give me the "answers" to what Little Lauren's past feelings and experiences were, the conversation between us, appertaining to why she no longer remembered, would be revelatory.

As the interview continued, we discussed my inability to connect with Little Lauren and my concern that, if I could not, then it would have a negative emotional impact on me and my clients. My play therapist, having also suffered childhood sexual abuse, had great insights into the difficulties faced by wounded healers whose past traumas go unresolved. I had always believed that her experiences were an integral part of her work, allowing her to connect with me on a deeper level. Landreth (2012) recognises the active role that play therapists must take, both emotionally and physically. He also voices that "the therapist is also affected by the person of the child and the relationship" (Landreth, 2012: 111); what if the person affected is not the adult but the once wounded child within the therapist? I was attempting to avoid exposing Little Lauren to the hurt of my clients but, as I sat in front of my fabulous wounded healer, my thoughts turned to how this exposure had affected her.

*How I described me in the playroom is that I always felt that I took her in and said, "there you go; there is another one to inform me of", and that she (her 'inner child') . . . the impact on her . . . I was very aware of. But mine was very disassociated. She couldn't be with me any other time and I just had to do a piece of work to let her go. I can't stand the pain. . . . I had to think, "is this right? To keep on abusing my inner child". . . . Or should I let her go and let her be free?*

(Play Therapist Interview, March 2017)

Taking her "inner child" into the playroom made her, in my opinion, a fantastic therapist, but meant that her inner child was abused over and over again in the process: the child and adult remained separate, dissociated from one another. She was a crusader for others, but at a cost to herself.

*There was nothing left of me to give anybody anymore.*

(Play Therapist Interview, March 2017)

Freeing that child, as she has, later in life, allowed her to integrate her experiences and claim the voice of her inner child in recognition of the fact that it was not sustainable for her to be the hero for all children at the expense of herself. I too wish to be a voice for the voiceless; I know that doing this and also having a long and happy career entails the incorporation of Little Lauren into the fullness of my being and the rejection of the dissociation that for many years I welcomed in order to avoid pain. In interview, my play therapist also revealed that this journey of self-discovery and understanding would last for the rest of my life but that, in the process, I would leave the "monsters" behind and be the person and therapist that I chose to be in the present.

Van der Kolk (2014) and Janet (1925) cite the potential harm that stifling memories through dissociation can have. Personally, the most effective means of reconnecting with memory and acknowledging invisible demons was writing: it allowed me to express myself, free from the judgement of others (Van der Kolk, 2014). I could then implement the autoethnographic technique of holding these written "fragments of life against the present light and [make] sense of their significance within the bigger context of my life" (Chang, 2013: 115). My attempts at connecting with the part of me that I had consciously set adrift were initially futile: no connection could be made. Subsequently, when I began to connect viscerally with my younger self through therapeutic written exercises, I began to regain my sense of self. I was engulfed by sensations, memories and emotions of the past. For the first time I could see why being called "brave" had always provoked such a negative response in me: It was because Little Lauren had not felt brave for disclosing. She had felt victimised, angry and other-than. I could see that the anger I felt towards my father was not the 26-year-old's anger but the nine-year-old girl's anger at her father for not being her hero. Through engagement in a dialogue with my younger self, I felt like I was letting her go from the prison of the past, incorporating her into my present, and letting her know it would be alright. I view children's ability to disclose their abusive experiences as brave and I can finally say that Little Lauren was brave; I am brave. It was me, "I was abused" and I am breaking the silence of the awful isolation this imparts.

---

- It's not fair.
  - *I know.*
- But it's not fair!
  - *It's not. It never was.*
- It's alright for you! You're not here. You aren't feeling what I'm feeling. You are ok.
  - *I do. I have felt what you are feeling. I know how sad you are. I have felt the rage bubbling under the surface. I have stood in your shoes. I have lost what you have lost. I know that you are scared. I know how guilty you feel. But I know how strong and brave you are. You are going to be alright.*
- DON'T CALL ME BRAVE! I HATE IT!
  - *I know you do. I hate it too but it's true.*
- Being brave doesn't stop all this though! It doesn't stop it happening! It doesn't stop them leaving. It doesn't stop mum and dad falling apart. I have ruined everything.
  - *I know it feels like that, but you will be ok.*
- Will I be messed up?
  - *NO. You won't. Not at all. You will feel out of control for a while, but everything will be fine. In fact, you'll be proud of who you'll become.*
- What about mum and dad?
  - *Ok. Well, dad isn't going to handle this well. He is going to struggle. He is going to say things he doesn't mean because he is hurting too. You are going to get mad. You are going to get so angry that you aren't going to know what to do. You are going to want to scream and cry and punch the bed so hard that it will scare you. Do it. It's ok. For a while you are going to feel like you hate him, but this will change. It will pass. It gets better. You'll laugh with him again and you will be proud that he is your dad.*

- And mum?

  - *She is going to struggle too but she will be ok. Go easy on her. You are going to want to give her all your problems, your upset, but you'll have to wait a while until she's stronger. But mum, well . . . she is mum. She is going to be your best friend. She is going to let you get away with murder sometimes, but you'll never take the mick. She will always be there for you. She will never let you down. Do me a favour and tell her how much you love her when you hit your teens.*

- I will.

  - *You'll be ok. We are just a normal girl. A normal, brilliant, brave girl.*

- Thank you.

                              (Therapeutic writing exercise, February 2017)

I cried as I wrote and, with each word, a new understanding of how I felt, and why, was achieved. It allowed me to claim my voice and has given me strength to help others without re-traumatising my younger self in the process. Little Lauren can still inform me about aspects of children's behaviour but in a controlled, incorporated and thoughtful way. She is a part of me and always will be.

When I enter into work with clients, experiencing difficulties that I too faced as a child, I have learnt to be particularly mindful. Countertransference can often occur and this must be worked through and addressed within supervision and personal therapy. I have also had to think about my approach. I am aware that what was therapeutically right for me as a child may not be right for others. I have given the issue of self-disclosure particular attention. My therapist's self-disclosure was extremely positive for me, but I have resolved that I would not be comfortable using this approach so overtly within my own practice. I do not feel that my clients would benefit from knowing details about my own abusive experiences and would fear that it would place a burden of responsibility and worry on them. I have, however, experienced the positive impact that addressing my own woundedness in a non-specific way with clients can have (Zerubavel & O'Dougherty Wright, 2012). Gaines (2003) discusses child therapists' use of self-disclosure as a means of displaying their own personality and, thus, promoting therapeutic communication. He also suggests that the therapist's willingness to reveal of themselves as the child does, and their readiness to disclose their conflicts and failures, as an idolised adult, can be of tremendous help in aiding the child's healing (Gaines, 2003).

Children often seek reassurances that they are not 'alone' in their experiences. They will inquire, "has something like this happened to you?", testing that I am someone who will understand. I will answer such questions with, "when I was little I had difficult times too" or "I felt similar hurts and fears when I was young". This non-specific disclosure allows the child to see the wounded healer duality that exists within me and, I hope, will give them confidence that recovery is possible (Zerubavel & O'Dougherty Wright, 2012). I also find that my willingness to share a little of my own woundedness redistributes the power imbalance that can often exist between adult and child. It is not only the child who is expected to be truly authentic and open, but me also. This cultivates feelings of safety, openness and valuable sharing of experiences, whilst lessening feelings of stigma and "otherness" that abused children often experience.

## The three of us

It is accepted that parents/carers are an integral part of the total therapeutic experience. Their support and close engagement with the play therapist can enable the child to experience the maximum benefit of therapy and act as a vehicle to heal strained or difficult relationships (McGuire & McGuire, 2001). We must, however, recognise that parents/carers will, naturally, have a "myriad of feelings about bringing their child to play therapy" (McGuire & McGuire, 2001: 17): shame, fear, reluctance, hope, anxiety, excitement, anger. These feelings can fluctuate over the course of the therapeutic process as time, circumstances, understandings, perspectives and coping strategies change and evolve. Thus, meeting with the parents at regular intervals is essential for the therapist. It ensures the parent/ carers are involved and "provides an opportunity for parental feedback regarding developmental progress and emotional/behavioural change" (Landreth, 2012: 132). As such, important partners in the play therapy process, we, as therapists, must give careful consideration to how we view and work with parents in our professional capacity. Conducting reflexive-dyadic interviews with my parents during my autoethnographic research project awakened me to new viewpoints regarding my own process and also gave me insights into the play therapy process as experienced by parents. Eliciting the perspectives of my parents created a co-constructed narrative of my childhood therapeutic journey in its fullness. It helped to show multiple perspectives of the same epiphany, exploring separate stories and reactions, and then assembling them into one collective account (Ellis et al., 2011). My story has always involved others. In my role of researcher and with my "researcher's eye", I observed things and learnt facts that would have gone unnoticed or unknown in my role as "daughter".

Bromfield (1992: 46) describes how "entrusting your child to any caretaker is hard. Entrusting your child to a therapist, and to the vulnerability of treatment is even harder". My play therapy sessions were a cherished and confidential space away from my parents and others. In my day-to-day life I would sometimes feel suffocated by the seemingly constant need of my parents to talk about and analyse what had happened and how I was feeling. Following my disclosure of abuse, I did not want anything in my life to change, I just wanted the abuse to stop. However, within days of my disclosure, the police and social services were involved and many of my family members took a stance that made continued contact impossible. I felt a total lack of control and my play therapy sessions allowed me some distance and time in which to process my complicated feelings. I could be vulnerable with my play therapist in a way that I could not with my parents; I did not fear upsetting her as I did them. I viewed them as fragile; it was my belief that I was to blame for their pain. My parents had been the ones to seek out therapeutic support for me and were always very vocal in their support of the process; they understood that I needed a private space, away from them, in order to begin to heal. My reality had always been that, as a family, our perception of play therapy was wholly positive. In interviews, however, I learnt that there were aspects of the play therapy process that had been deeply painful for them.

> *You became distant . . . in a way. You were empowered by your play therapist and it changed how you thought and how you were and you worked through that with her and you didn't want to talk through it so much with me.*
> *(Mother Interview, March 2017)*

Before therapy, our relationship was one of openness and I was very dependent on her. Now, at age nine, I had another woman with whom I also shared some of my most intimate and exposing thoughts and feelings (through words and play). This time was confidential and "unknown" to my mother. The power and importance of the therapeutic relationship were not something that had been discussed with her prior to my therapy starting; nor did my mother feel comfortable enough to share her feelings of powerlessness with my therapist. She trusted that my therapist was the "expert" in their dynamic and that she did not have the answers. Landreth (2001: 89) recognises 'that the issue of confidentiality can be difficult for some parents'; they are accustomed to being the adults responsible for the child, responsible for finding solutions to problems for that child. My mother certainly found entrusting this role to my therapist challenging. Discovering this made me reflect on the way I work with parents. I felt I needed to scrutinise my practice and consider lessening the feelings of powerlessness for parents. I believe that the biggest catalyst for positive change in therapists' relationships with parents is the therapist's attitude and outlook. If parents are to collaborate in the therapeutic process, we must listen to them fully and attempt to understand their viewpoints and foster feelings of honesty and respect (Landreth, 2001). The difficult feelings that the confidential nature of therapy can trigger for parents is something I discuss openly. I also feel it necessary to give parents time and a listening ear so they can verbalise and explore their feelings without judgement. This approach recognises and facilitates their "potential to learn, to explore themselves, and to grow" (Landreth, 2001: 85).

In my work with families, I can also find myself questioning decisions made by parents, or find it hard to see the child in the playroom reflected in their descriptions. It is at this point that I must be mindful and remind myself of what I tell parents during our initial meeting; "you are the expert on your child". I see their child for one hour per week and, if my own time in play therapy is anything to go by, the child may not always show me the more negative aspects of their behaviour. Parents are often with the child seven days a week and experience the highs, lows and everything in between. Landreth (2001: 86) posits that we must therefore work "together with parents by making suggestions, asking for ideas, and together determining what is effective". This will lessen feelings of powerlessness and will instead give them the confidence that they have the resources to support their child, not only whilst they are having therapy, but for the rest of their lives.

Interviews with my parents aided my remembering of events from the past. When I thought about my time in play therapy, I only recalled snippets of my one-to-one sessions. However, when my parents and I began to discuss my experiences in more depth, I was reminded of review meetings, when we had all been involved. My memories of these were mostly negative and, as I spoke about them in the present, with the two people who had endured them with me, I was reminded of how upsetting, confusing and frustrating they had been for us all.

As previously mentioned, meeting with parents at regular intervals in order to keep them engaged in the process is essential, something I do every six to eight weeks within my own clinical practice, their structure heavily informed by my own childhood experiences of review meetings and their emotional impact. I believe that review meetings should not be conducted with the child in attendance (apart from in special circumstances); these consultations allow parents to be frank regarding their thoughts and feelings about the child and/or their behaviours, or the situation that has brought them to therapy which could be harmful and/or inappropriate for the child to hear. I also use review meetings as an opportunity to briefly train parents in skills that will aid them in responding to their child in a more positive way (Landreth, 2012). These include such skills as reflecting feelings, limit setting and self-esteem-boosting exercises, giving choice and modelling behaviours. As review meetings are mainly with the parent/s, I ensure that I inform the child that the meeting will be taking place and ask if there is anything they would like me to discuss or feedback to the parent. At the start of the following session, I then take five to ten minutes to discuss the outcome of the review meeting and answer questions. This maintains honesty and congruence within the therapeutic relationship, lessens anxieties and still allows the child a voice in the meeting.

My childhood review meetings were conducted with all present: me, my mother, my father and my play therapist. My therapist's feedback regarding my progress, struggles and difficulties with aspects of my parents' behaviours and reactions towards me were discussed in my presence. As a family, we were then encouraged, with the support of my therapist, to find solutions, compromises and responses that would support my well-being. In theory, this could have been an exercise that brought us together and helped to heal some of the hurt that existed between us. What had been overlooked was that we were all at very different stages emotionally. We might as well have been speaking different languages. Both my mother and father echoed this sentiment during interview:

> *My abiding memory of the three of us sitting there is that we were all talking in different ways about things. There was no . . . I just remember sitting there and just thinking we are not connected. Not properly connected with this. We haven't all got the same understanding of this.*
>
> (Mother Interview, March 2017)

> *. . . in other words, you know, at a fraction of my age, it was almost like you had come to terms with something that I couldn't come to terms with.*
>
> (Father's Interview, March 2017)

My relationship with my father was the most strained and difficult and suggestions were made by my therapist to help us communicate better: acknowledging each other's feelings, breathing exercises to help us to remain calm, and shared activities. My father seemed to understand these suggestions and was insistent that he would follow them through; I felt hopeful and expectant of success. When we tried to implement this into our day-to-day lives, the reality was very different. My father did not have the foundational understanding to support me in my emotional adjustment as these positive factors were absent in his own childhood experiences of parenting. He was also suffering from PTSD impairing his emotional responses. At the age of nine, I was not able to intellectualise and understand the reasons for his inabilities in this vein, instead it hurt me deeply and exacerbated my feelings of low self-worth. I believed that I was unlovable and not worthy of his efforts. This fuelled my anger and only intensified the distance between us. I was also comparing my therapist's emotional responses to his. The contrast was so stark that I simply could not understand why he had no grasp of my internal world. My anger and frustration resulted in the need to distance myself from my parents for a time; their lack of understanding was keeping me stuck.

> *What I feel . . . is that you had to separate yourself from us as your parents for a while. It enabled you to become resilient . . . as we were keeping you stuck in a place, you no longer wanted, or needed to be. To me I think this was because we all healed at different times. With hindsight you were protecting yourself as a child in an instinctual way; especially as both dad and myself are too prone to intellectualise hurt, when all you needed was to feel protected and safe.*
>
> (Mothers Interview, November 2019)

It has taken many years of work and self-reflection for myself and my father to heal the emotional wounds inflicted upon each other and I do believe that my review meetings were a hindrance rather than a help in this. Landreth (2012) suggests a parent of a child in play therapy should also be in therapy themselves. I believe that, in the majority of cases, the parent receiving therapeutic support alongside their child could only be advantageous; as Landreth (2012: 128) states, "when parents feel better about themselves, are less anxious, and are better adjusted, they are more likely to respond in positive, self-enhancing ways to their children". I strongly believe that we have a duty of care to our clients to protect them from harm through the most rigorous consideration, case by case, we can employ.

## Concluding thoughts

*I am sat in front of my laptop, and I feel stuck.*
*I remember the feeling. It is the same feeling I had when I tried to summa-*
*    rise my dissertation.*
*I am sat here wanting to type. Needing to type. Yet my fingers are not willing.*
*Is it because I simply do not have anything to say? No . . . it's the opposite.*
*    I feel OVERWHELMED. Overwhelmed with the enormity of it. How do*
*    I conclude something that has not yet concluded?*
*How do I conclude a process that is ever changing?*
                              (Therapeutic Writing Exercise, August 2020)

"Conclusion" is defined as "the end or finish of an event, process, or text" (Stevenson, 2010: 362). It is easy to summarise texts in a contained format with a clear beginning, middle and end. My personal process of play therapy is much harder to conclude as it does not have a finite ending, nor shape. This is because, as Landreth (2012: 104) wrote, a "therapist is a real person, not a robot". I am complex, with my own thoughts, motivations, needs and ways of relating to the world around me and these actions are influenced and impacted upon by my memories and experiences. It can be said that one's "self" does not remain static and we must be alert and responsive to these shifts within ourselves, constantly open to change and adaption. My status as "wounded healer" dictates that I engage in continual self-exploration, both professionally and socially, minimising the potential for my own needs and motivations to impact my clients, and enabling my own continued healing of existing wounds. However, this does not have to be a torturous task; rather, it is a way of being in the world that "requires living consciously, emotionally, reflexively" (Ellis, 2013: 10). I learnt this way of "being" through engaging with the autoethnographic process, a process that I found life changing. It taught me that examining my own life is not enough, I must also consider how and why I think and act in the ways that I do (Ellis, 2013). It also opened my eyes to the idea of multiple "selves" being contained within a singular self, each existing in different times and contexts and each with their own voice. These differing "selves" never appear to exist in isolation but instead inform each other, engaging in a continual inner dialogue that enlightens and educates me in the present.

I have learnt a great deal through my self-exploration and not all can be contained within this brief overview. What I have learnt, however, has positively impacted my therapeutic work and, I hope, could provoke thought in those who read this chapter. My childhood experiences of play therapy, and later interactions with my childhood play therapist, speak to the need for therapists to enter into the therapeutic relationship with solidness, resilience and the warm reassurance that healing and recovery are possible; that we will stand with them in the darkness instead of shying away from their pain. It also reminds us that, although our own wounds can provide insight, "wounded healers" must take particular care not to "give all" to others at a cost to themselves. This is a fact that was evidenced by my play therapist's burnout and is consistently confirmed by researchers' studies of compassion fatigue, finding "that wounded healers are more vulnerable than other therapists to being traumatised by the clinical work itself" (Zerubavel & O'Dougherty Wright, 2012: 484).

As a play therapist it is my role to support children and families in their healing and growth, both as individuals and collectively. I believe it is imperative that the therapeutic relationship is grounded in the belief that recovery and a bright future are achievable. This is not to say that, once therapy is ended, clients will not experience struggles and difficulties but that we should hope to equip them with the strategies and emotional resilience to better cope when those instances arise. Parents/carers act as a keystone for equipping their children with this long-term resilience. Although we must give parent/carers the tools and understanding to help support their children long after therapy has ended, we must also be open and honest: recovery is not always linear, but this fact should not be feared. My mother often told me, after my play therapy ended, that my therapist had confided that significant life events (e.g. entering into relationships, marriage, motherhood) may trigger potentially complex or negative emotional responses or feelings that would require examination and emotional strength. Awareness of this conversation in regard to this potential was a valuable insight, and strangely comforting, in relation to significant rites of passage. My response to complex inner dialogues at these times was "normal". Clearly, the experiences and learning I have described had equipped me with the emotional understanding, tools and strength to remain present in the here and now, whilst making conscious decisions about who and how I wished to be. Self-discovery and understanding is a life-long process, a process I am committed to pursuing with great optimism and no small measure of excitement.

## References

Adams, E. & Holman Jones, S. (2008) Autoethnography is Queer. In   Denzin, N. K., Lincoln, Y. S. & Smith, L. T. (eds.) *Handbook of Critical and Indigenous Methodologies* (pp. 373–390). Thousand Oaks, CA: Sage.

Aponte, H. & Winter, J. (1987) *The Person and Practice of the Therapist: Treatment and Training.* In: Baldwin, B. & Satir, V. (eds.) *The Use of Self in Therapy* (pp. 85–111). London: The Haworth Press.

Axline, V. (1969) *Play Therapy.* New York: Ballantine Books.

Barnett, M. (2007) What Brings You Here? An Exploration of the Unconscious Motivations of Those Who Choose to Train and Work as Psychotherapists and Counsellors. *Psychodynamic Practice,* 13(3), pp. 257–274.

Beitchman, J., Zucker, K., Hood, J. & DaCosta, G. (1992) A Review of the Long-Term Effects of Child Sexual Abuse. *Child Abuse and Neglect,* 16(1), pp. 101–118.

Braham, J. (1995) *Crucial Conversations: Interpreting Contemporary American Literary Autobiography of Women.* New York: Teachers College Press.

Briere, J. & Elliott, D. (1994) Immediate and Long-Term Impacts of Child Sexual Abuse. *The Future of Children,* 4(2), pp. 54–69.

Bromfield, R. (1992) *Playing for Real: The World of a Play Therapist.* New York: Dutton.

Cattanach, A. (2008) *Play Therapy With Abused Children* (2nd ed.). London: Jessica Kingsley Publishers.

Chang, H. (2013) *Individual and Collaborative Autoethnography as Method.* In: Jones, S., Adams, T. & Ellis, C. (eds.) *Handbook of Autoethnography* (pp. 107–122). New York: Routledge.

Christensen, E. (2011) *The Construction of Self in an Adult Survivor of Childhood Sexual Abuse.* PHD Thesis. University of New Orleans. Available at: http://scholarworks.uno.edu/cgi/viewcontent.cgi?article=2279&context=td (Accessed: 2 February 2017).

Ellis, C. (2013) *Carrying the Torch for Autoethnography.* In: Jones, S., Adams, T. & Ellis, C. (ed.) *Handbook of Autoethnography* (pp. 9–12). New York: Routledge.

Ellis, C., Adams, T. & Bochner, A. (2011) *Autoethnography: An Overview,* 12(1) [40 paragraphs]. Available at: www.qualitative-research.net/index.php/fqs/article/view/1589/3095 (Accessed: 5 January 2017).

Farber, B. A., Manevich, I., Metzger, J. & Saypol, E. (2005) Choosing Psychotherapy as a Career: Why Did We Cross That Road? *Journal of Clinical Psychology,* 61(8), pp. 1009–1031.

Gefter, J., Bankoff, S., Valentine, E., Rood, B. & Pantalone, W. (2013) Feminist Beliefs Associated With Young Women's Recovery From Male-Perpetrated Abuse. *Women and Therapy,* 36, pp. 332–355.

Gaines, R. (2003) Therapist Self-Disclosure With Children, Adolescents, and Their Parents. *Journal of Clinical Psychology,* 59(5), pp. 569–580.

Gil, E. (1991) *The Healing Power of Play: Working With Abused Children.* London: Guilford Press.

Gordon Clark, L. (2019) *Training Issues: Before, During and After.* In: Ayling, P., Armstrong, H. & Gordon Clark, L. (eds.) *Becoming and Being a Play Therapist: Play therapy in Practice* (pp. 11–23). London: Routledge.

Holman-Jones, S. (2005) Auto Ethnography: Making the Personal Political. In: Denzin, N. K. and Lincoln, Y. S. (eds.) *Handbook of Qualitative Research* (pp. 763–791), Thousand Oaks: Sage.

Janet, P. (1925) *Psychological Healing.* New York: Macmillan.

Jennings, S. (1993) *Play Therapy With Children: A Practitioner's Guide.* Oxford: Blackwell Scientific.

Landreth, G. (ed.). (2001) *Innovations in Play Therapy: Issues, Process, and Special Populations.* New York: Brunner-Routledge.

Landreth, G. (2012) *Play Therapy: The Art of the Relationship*. New York: Routledge.

Lanyado, M. (2004) *The Presence of the Therapist: Treating Childhood Trauma*. East Sussex: Brunner-Routledge.

Metta, M. (2010) *Writing Against, Alongside and Beyond Memory*. Oxford: Peter Lang Publishing.

McAdams, D. (2006) The Problem of Narrative Coherence. *Journal of Constructivist Psychology*, 19(2), pp. 109–125.

McGuire, D. K. & McGuire, D. E. (2001) *Linking Parents to Play therapy: A Practical Guide With Applications, Interventions, and Case Studies*. Lillington, NC: Taylor & Francis.

Putnam, F. (2003) Ten-Year Research Update Review: Child Sexual Abuse. *Academy of Child and Adolescent Psychiatry*, 43(3), 269–278.

Satir, V. (1987) The Therapists Story. *Journal of Psychotherapy and the Family*. 3(1), 17–25. Taylor Francis Online.

Scott, S. (2001) Surviving Selves: Feminism and Contemporary Discourse of Child Sexual Abuse. *Feminist Theory*, 2(3), pp. 349–361.

Spry, T. (2001) Performing Autoethnography: An Embodied Methodological Praxis. *Qualitative Inquiry*, 7(6), pp. 706–732.

Stevenson, A. (2010) *Oxford Dictionary of English* (3rd ed.). Oxford: Oxford University Press.

Van der Kolk, B. (2014) *The Body Keeps the Score: Mind, Brain and Body in the Transformation of Trauma*. London: Penguin Random House.

Yalom, I. D. (1985) *The Theory and Practice of Group Psychotherapy* (3rd ed.). New York: Basic Books.

Zerubavel, N. & O'Dougherty-Wright, M. (2012) The Dilemma of the Wounded Healer. *American Psychological Association*, 49(4), pp. 482–491.

# Chapter 4

# A hero's journey

## Finding gold at the end of the rainbow

*Sarah Zehetmayr-McCall*
*and Lisa Gordon Clark*

### Chapter overview

This chapter will provide an overview of my personal process of being a bereaved play therapist working within a bereavement service, and it will also reflect on these processes within the clinical supervisor/supervisee relationship. Clinical supervision has been an essential activity in aiding me to deepen my understanding of my *Self*, in particular my bereavement experience, and the impact grief can have on the therapeutic relationship between the child and the therapist. As a play therapist, it is imperative to work in a safe and ethical manner in order to minimise a play therapist's personal process being played out within the therapeutic relationship, undermining the heart of the therapeutic work, and potentially causing harm to the child.

I will discuss several clinical issues explored within supervision, using vignettes to illustrate the challenges and opportunities I faced as a play therapist who continues to grieve the death of her eldest child. I will explore what triggers my grief, including rainbows, ambulances, death and dying play, Christmas, and the subsequent psychosocial difficulties and somatic experiences I have when my personal grief is present within the therapeutic relationship. These issues were discussed within the clinical supervisor/supervisee relationship I formed with Lisa Gordon Clark in 2017. Lisa, as my clinical supervisor, has contributed in a positive way to my ability to openly discuss my personal process, and the parallel processes that can happen, within the therapeutic relationship (Henderson et al., 2014). This has been an essential activity for developing a conscious awareness of my *Self* in my capacity as a play therapist. Furthermore, my grief is not an event but rather an ongoing process needing diligent attention, through continued engagement with clinical supervision, to ensure it does not interfere with a child's need to explore their own journey of loss, sadness and hope.

*Lisa: Interspersed through Sarah's chapter I will add some brief comments on my perspective of her process and my role within it as her clinical supervisor. These will be italicised to differentiate my voice from hers for the reader.*

DOI: 10.4324/9781003017271-4

## Introduction

The death of a loved one leaves one irrevocably changed, but it does not necessarily mean there is no hope of healing or finding gifts from grief and sorrow (Levine, 2005; Harris, 2020; Nouwen, 2014; Rosenberg, 2015). As someone who has been through the death of a child, I have found that every fibre of my mind and body has changed. My grief brings me great sadness, and yet maybe surprisingly, there have also been gifts of joy at the same time. For me, it has become a "Hero's Journey" (Lahad, 1997), knowing that when there is both sunshine and showers, there is the possibility of a rainbow and, although elusive, when the fragmented light becomes one, there is always the hope of a pot of gold at the end of it. In 1949, mythologist Joseph Campbell (2008) published *The Hero with a Thousand Faces*, which outlines the structure of the journeys that archetypical heroes experience in world myths. This structure became known as the monomyth, or Hero's Journey, and has since served as the framework behind many popular fiction books and films, including *Star Wars, Harry Potter and the Sorcerer's Stone* and *The Lord of the Rings*. I have found the symbolism of rainbows has resonated throughout my grieving process: rainbows are symbolic in many cultures as a bridge between heaven and earth, and as promise of hope (Chevalier & Gheerbrant, 1996). Furthermore, in my play therapy work with bereaved children I have found rainbows to be a reoccurring theme and symbol of hope emerging out of children's grief. My own *Hero's Journey* has not come to an end as yet; I continue to grieve; it is a life-long journey (Lahad, 1997). Nouwen (2014: 87) suggests "making our [*own*] wounds available as a source for healing". My own grief and wounds are present with me every day, and with every bereaved child I work with as a play therapist. It is the knowledge of the depths of grief, loss and hope in my own personal process that underpins my play therapy work, all the while ensuring that it does not overshadow or indeed prevent the child's own *Hero's Journey* to shine through.

I have found it can be difficult and exhausting to hold the child's grief and my own grief simultaneously. Yet, my personal process informs me, gives me insight and understanding of some of the feelings and thoughts bereaved children may experience and present within their play. However, I acknowledge the risk in the parallel processes and, at times, these may have led me to overidentify by only viewing children's play through the lens of bereavement, for example all burying of objects in the sand being directly linked to the death of a loved one. Through clinical supervision I have been able to harness the power of my personal experiences, allowing the child's process to be the focus of my attention without my own processes, biases and prejudices getting in the way and interfering with the child's (McMahon, 1992; Nouwen, 2014). Furthermore, clinical supervision has become central to my practice enabling me to manage and maintain my ability to name and know my *Self* (Rothschild, 2006; Yasenik & Gardner, 2012). Without this understanding I believe my capacity to continue to work in the field of bereavement would have been greatly reduced due to the risk of secondary trauma

(Cattanach, 2008; Macran & Shapiro, 1998; Perry, 2014). Through clinical supervision I have learned how to better contain my personal processes, and to recognise how *Self* may impact on the therapeutic relationship, whilst also not denying nor cutting myself off from my own bereavement experience. This ensures not only my safe and ethical practice as a play therapist but enables me to continue to support bereaved children in the here and now, and hopefully, long into the future.

This chapter is not a chapter about bereavement or clinical supervision per se. Rather, it is about the importance of knowing oneself intimately through clinical supervision for the purpose of practising in a safe and ethical manner (BAPT, 2021). As already noted, personal experiences can be useful when working in a setting, which provides play therapy to those with similar experiences to one's own, including hypothesising about children's processes (Stone, 2019; Worden, 2003). However, these hypotheses need to be carefully considered within the clinical supervision relationship in order not to jump to conclusions which have been skewed by one's own perspective. As Ryan and Wilson (2000: 157) note, a therapist may sometimes need help in supervision to avoid overstepping "her professional role . . . (and) in refraining from overpersonalising her already close relationship with the child", and I believe this is particularly the case when there are parallel experiences. At times, in clinical supervision, I have had to dig deep to be open, vulnerable and reflect on the deeply personal and traumatic experience of my own child's death. In personal therapy I have examined the trauma of this bereavement. However, it is in clinical supervision where I have been able to explore and acknowledge triggers and flashbacks within the context of the therapeutic relationship, and the hypotheses I make about bereaved children's play. To enable their supervisees to feel safe enough to do this essential reflection, clinical supervisors need to provide genuineness, warmth and unconditional positive regard much like the therapist/client relationship (Rogers, 1957). I believe without Rogers' core conditions in place I would only have engaged with clinical supervision at a superficial level, therefore never getting to the heart of my own personal process, and the subsequent parallel processes. McMahon (1992) argues that working therapeutically with children is difficult and at times painful work. A therapist's own traumas may rise to the surface, and therefore it is crucial for therapists to develop self-awareness and the ability to separate their personal process from that of the child's (McCann, 2019; Worden, 2003). Without the safe place of supervision, I would be at risk not only of cutting myself off from my grief, but also of denying the gifts grief has brought me, such as greater insight and knowledge of loss and bereavement (Levine, 2005; Rosenberg, 2015; Rothschild, 2006). This parallel process of holding both the positive and negative aspects of one's own journey along with another person's grief mirrors healthy grieving. Stroebe and Schut (1999) argue that in order for a grieving person to develop resilience they need to be able to move backwards and forwards between the dual aspects of grieving, that is the grief-orientated and restoration-orientated loss processes. Furthermore, if I were to have poor self-awareness, at best I might deny the child's personal process of loss, transformation and hope, but at worst,

I might cause significant psychosocial and emotional harm to an already vulnerable child (Daniels & Jenkins, 2010; Macran & Shapiro, 1998; McMahon, 1992; Rose, 2012).

*From the outset, clinical supervision sessions together were characterised by Sarah's openness and an impressive level of self-awareness as she began to share the profound personal experiences of the past that informed her practice in the present. It was hugely helpful for her therapeutic practice that she was able to confront her feelings head-on and was willing to acknowledge and explore her struggles within the containment of supervision.*

*Her process notes, reliably sent to me in advance of each supervision session, were a testament to her diligence and to her reflective capacity. The right-hand column, where she considered themes of the child's work and her responses to them, was always insightful, open and constructive. She was not afraid to acknowledge when she had struggled, to admit when she was anxious, but also increasingly to note when she felt hopeful, experienced warm feelings and when she shifted gear. One set of process notes summarises her impressions from "feeling positive" at the start, noticing some anxiety creeping in, feeling deeply sad, but also "in awe of the child", and culminating in feeling pleased with a sense of hopefulness in the child's abilities, resourcefulness, resilience and willingness to engage and trust her. She conceded that sometimes at first, she struggled to reflect the deeper meanings and feelings behind behaviour, but the more she was able to reflect on the deeper meanings and feelings behind her <u>own</u> responses, the more effective her practice became. That reflective capacity will become evident as this chapter unfolds.*

## The life changing event

In sharing my own *Hero's Journey* of finding gold at the end of the rainbow, I need to start at the beginning and provide some context to my bereavement. Andrew is my first born of three children. He loved trains, and we adored him. On Christmas day morning, we went to wake him, to tell him Father Christmas had been, only to find he had died some time in the night while he slept. He was aged 23 months and 5 days. Later, it was discovered that Andrew died from the H1N1 virus, Swine Flu, with no preceding symptoms or known underlying health conditions. I have my life before and my life after Andrew's death. My life hinges on this day. The loss and devastation of Andrew's death are an integral part of who I am and what I have become. In amongst the trauma and chaos of that day, and the days that followed, Christmas festivities continued in the world around me and my family, whilst ours felt like it had come to a grinding halt. For others, Christmas went on, presents were given and unwrapped, there was the eating of the Christmas turkey, and families celebrating their "togetherness". All the while, our world had become a very dark, lonely and frightening place. There seemed to be no hope, no room for happiness and no life beyond that day. Yet the next day I chose to live, to move forward, by making the simplest but hardest of steps by getting out of bed. There have been days I have returned to bed and "hidden" under the duvet. Nevertheless, I have continued to make my way forward, travelling with Andrew forever in my heart. He is the reason I began working in a bereavement setting and eventually became a play therapist.

## Life before bereavement

In writing this chapter on the personal process of being a bereaved play therapist working in a bereavement setting, I need to acknowledge being bereaved is not all of whom or what I am. I had a life before my life became defined by the death of Andrew. It was a life not without its own struggles and challenges. I am a woman who has experienced childhood medical and educational trauma due to congenital disability and dyslexia. Professionals had low expectations of me and my future. However, I come from a family of fighters and high achievers. My parents owned a care home for older people, and we lived above "the shop". Consequently, I have always had death and dying as part of my life. It was not uncommon for conversations about *so and so* dying to take place around the family dinner table, after all they were part of the family. These experiences, and being a practising Christian, resulted in me wanting to help and support other vulnerable people and I qualified as a social worker in 2001. Having reflected over the years on my early childhood experiences of trauma, the normalisation of death and dying, my faith, and working as a social worker, I recognise that all these experiences have equipped me with the emotional resources and resilience for when Andrew died.

## Being a bereaved play therapist

Since 2014, I have worked in an adult hospice, in my capacity as a social worker, with children and families who have experienced the death of a significant family member. I only began my training to become a play therapist in 2015. This type of work can be difficult and challenging for anyone, and maybe more so for me as my own grief can be triggered daily. Worden (2003) and Sawyer (2015) both warn that those working within palliative care settings need to be vigilant and ensure they practise adequate self-care, as it is emotionally demanding work with a high risk of burnout. One way of practising self-care is by increasing self-awareness through clinical supervision. Ray (2011) argues that it is within clinical supervision that the supervisee can become more congruent through this process of heightened self-awareness, which is central to the development of the therapeutic relationship. Landreth (2012) states that without the necessary clinical supervision, and it must be said personal therapy, therapists are in danger of burnout, especially when working with children who have experienced such challenging life events. In considering all this, it could be argued that for me personally and professionally, becoming a play therapist may well have been my saving grace. As a bereaved social worker, practising therapeutic play in a bereavement environment, I initially did not have the necessary support to deepen my understanding of my own personal issues and how these may impact on both the child and on myself. However, there is a balance to be struck between the exploration of the therapist's experience and needs, against that of their clients; therefore, supervisors may need to support supervisees to engage in personal therapy (Lahad, 2000; Platteuw, 2019; Ray, 2011).

*Alongside helping Sarah to reflect on the clinical material of her clients I remained alert to when this had particular resonance for her. Platteuw (2019: 51) makes the important point that one of the key roles of a supervisor is to be mindful of the supervisee's personal well-being:*

> *Although it is not the supervisor's role to be a therapist to the supervisee, inevitably personal issues impact on the supervisee's practice. Supervisors should be alive to such issues, be a nurturing presence and supportively reflect upon these, if appropriate, within supervision.*

*and that furthermore supervisors need to be alert to issues of secondary trauma (Perry, 2014). Secondary trauma is the stress resulting from helping, or wanting to help, a traumatised or suffering person and is sometimes referred to as Secondary Traumatic Stress (STS). This was also renamed "compassion fatigue" in 1995 by Charles Figley, who described it as the natural emotions that arise as a result of learning about a significant others' experience with a traumatic event or distress (Bercier & Maynard, 2015) and that lead to a reduced capacity to help. STS and compassion fatigue impact many individuals working in the mental health arena and there has been found to be a strong correlation between burnout and secondary traumatic stress among mental health care professionals who are indirectly exposed to trauma. I was aware that workers who have themselves had a history of trauma are particularly susceptible to developing STS. However, there are known protective factors against STS for mental health care workers, for example more time spent in self-care activities as well as high self-efficacy (Hensel et al., 2015), so in order to support Sarah and help her avoid burnout, I needed to ensure she looked after herself. Throughout her master's training of course this was complemented by regular personal therapy, but nevertheless there was always an important element of check-in on her well-being as part of our clinical supervision process. Indeed, this issue is so essential that Norcross and VandenBos (2018: 15) urged that clinicians "must make self-care a priority . . . Self-care is not a narcissistic luxury to be fulfilled as time permits; it is a human requisite, a clinical necessity, and an ethical imperative". Supervisors need to pay heed to this ethical imperative.*

Prior to becoming a play therapist, I recall a clinical issue I took to personal therapy, which had caused me distress as it had triggered my grief. A child had climbed into a large sky-blue sand tray and asked me to bury him, and his toy, in the sand. As he lay there with his legs and arms down by his side, with a serious look on his face, I had a flashback of Andrew, and *his* toy, having been laid out in his sky-blue coffin. I did not have the training, knowledge or the necessary play therapy clinical supervision at that time to know what to do with this child's process. Intuitively, I stayed with the child's play, despite my internal struggle, by acknowledging his request, although not acting on it. On reflection, I might have denied the child's personal process in not providing an alternative to burying him. This event still resonates with me today. As it was, I tried to sit with the child's process, yet felt deeply out of my depth, while holding my own traumatic memories at the same time (Worden, 2003). Even though Lisa was not my clinical supervisor at the time, this experience is something we have discussed on more than one occasion.

The above vignette reflects Yasenik and Gardner's (2012) insistence that therapists to know their *Self* before engaging in therapeutic work and for nurturing an ongoing reflective process to develop and increase self-awareness. Nouwen (2014) argues that through a willingness to be open to the pain of one's own grief, one can in turn help others to find healing from their own painful experience. Platteuw (2019) warns it is imperative to differentiate between client-focused supervision and personal issues. In clinical supervision, I have been able to explore both verbally and creatively the transference and countertransference of the therapeutic relationship. Clinical supervision has enabled me not only to protect the client from my own grief, but also to maintain my own health and emotional well-being, thereby protecting my longevity as a play therapist (Hawkins & Shohet, 2012).

## The formation of a clinical supervision relationship

Lisa and I formed a clinical supervision relationship in 2017 when I was undertaking my MSc in Play Therapy. To be honest, I was initially intimidated by the thought of being supervised by Lisa. I was worried my practice would be picked apart, that I would be criticised and harshly judged. My long-standing internal working model (Bowlby, 1973) of "you're not good enough" was ringing in my ears. However, nothing could have been further from the truth. Lisa was warm, caring, funny, humble and always curious. I looked forward to our fortnightly clinical supervision. In these sessions, I was able to peel back my conscious and unconscious personal processes being played out in the therapist/client relationship, while ensuring the client remained the focus of the supervisory relationship (Clarkson, 2003; Ray, 2011).

Hawkins and Shohet (2012) highlight how the therapist's countertransference, their responses and reactions to their client can provide insight into the client's world. In clinical supervision, I was able to explore the transference and countertransference between myself and my clients as well as my triggers and somatic experiences I would have during play therapy sessions. I work in a person-centred manner and I acknowledge I bring my whole *Self* to the therapeutic relationship and, therefore, Andrew is part of both my conscious and unconscious personal process, for Andrew cannot be left at the door of the play therapy room as I enter (Axline, 1969; Le Vay, 2016; Rogers, 1957; Stone, 2019; Yasenik & Gardner, 2012).

I must not only therapeutically hold the client in front of me but must also silently acknowledge Andrew's presence in my thoughts, feelings and mind. As I have become a more skilled play therapist, many of these thoughts and feelings remain unconscious and are safely held within myself. However, occasionally I am aware my own bereavement is triggered as a somatic experience, such as my mind wandering, becoming sleepy or having a heavy weight on my chest. To acknowledge this has taken courage and a willingness to be vulnerable, but that is nothing new to me – I am a survivor, like many of the children and families I have worked with. However, as a *Wounded Healer* (Nouwen, 2014) I needed a companion alongside me, to help me through my *Hero's Journey* safely and Lisa has fulfilled that role. Likewise, Lisa has facilitated me to become the trusted companion of many a bereaved child.

*When I first met Sarah at a British Association of Play Therapists (BAPT) conference in Spring 2017, I was immediately struck by her eager warmth and optimism but knew nothing of her back story and what had led her to train as a play therapist until after I had agreed to supervise her second year of training.*

*My notes of our first consultation in the August of that year record that she told me first of her congenital hip deformity which affects her mobility and impacts on her physical presence in the play therapy room. She spoke openly about the importance of addressing and naming this with children at the outset of her work, as she did with me. She went on to describe to me how she had had to "fight her way through life", leading her to possess lots of "tenacity". Then she calmly but poignantly told me about her three children and how Andrew's death was what had led her to bereavement work. She was transparent with me that "Andrew is often still in the room" and that her ongoing personal therapy was not just a course requirement, but an essential support in her own therapeutic work. I think we both shed a tear at the raw honesty of this.*

*My notes of that meeting also record that she was brave enough to admit to me her internal working model of "I am not worthy" and "I am not good enough" – in spite of having been awarded a distinction for most assignments in her training! As we got to know one another, we were able to joke often about this and about her high-achieving quest for perfection. Like many of my supervisees, and students, she needed help to accept that "good enough" (Winnicott, 1971) was indeed good enough. Actually, it soon became obvious she exceeded "good enough" by some margin!*

## Process of clinical supervision

I found being a play therapy student an intense personal and difficult experience for many reasons. However, having Lisa as my clinical supervisor has challenged me to aim higher and to achieve more. Therefore, I had to dig deeper than I realised I could, in order to know myself and develop my skills, knowledge and experience. As well as play therapy sessions having to be video recorded, I produced detailed and comprehensive play therapy process notes for clinical supervision.

Each time we met, Lisa would have read my process notes, and we would explore the seen, the unseen, the conscious and the unconscious processes of each play therapy session (Luff & Ingham, 1955). Together, we would review and analyse the video footage which greatly helped me not only to develop my knowledge and skills as a play therapist but also to deepen my self-awareness and self-understanding (Ray, 2011).

*Early on, I had to help Sarah manage her expectations of herself and had to be quite assertive when she was tempted to take on really complex cases, some involving significant developmental trauma, not straightforward bereavement work, which I could discern were inappropriate for a student placement. Sometimes one of the key roles for supervision in training (or in initial post-qualifying practice) is to be the voice of "no'" for an eager student who wants to be able to change the world. As a self-diagnosed "wounded healer" (Nouwen, 2014), Sarah wanted to heal the world, but this eagerness needed to be balanced by recognition of the limitations of her own still fledgling skills and minimal experience as a play therapist.*

*Although I do not adhere rigidly to any particular theoretical model of supervision, I have found it interesting to consider my supervisory relationship with Sarah in the light of the "Integrative developmental model of supervision" (Stoltenberg & McNeill, 2010). This delineates four different levels of progression beginning with the therapist being unsure of their clinical practice and seeking explicit guidance and teaching from their supervisor in order to hone their skills. Since, Sarah began with me halfway through her master's training, and because of her extensive prior experience as a social worker, I perceived that she was already fairly confident in her basic therapeutic skills and although she certainly valued guidance, she was quickly able to progress to level 2 and focus less on her own anxieties and more on the needs of her clients. Indeed, she moved quite swiftly on to level 3, where she demonstrated more autonomy, independent thinking and awareness of her response to different clients. In levels 3 and 3i, supervisees use their supervisors more in a consultancy role and this development transpired with Sarah when she took what she felt was the "brave step" of challenging my thinking as we watched together video footage of one of the episodes of play, she had brought to show me. Venturing to assert a different point of view suggests real trust in the safety of the supervisory relationship too and on my own part represents what I hope is a humble openness to new ideas and perspectives. I willingly acknowledge now that I learn almost as much from most of my experienced supervisees as they do from me.*

## Introduction to vignettes

The following vignettes provided in this chapter have all been chosen because a child's play process has triggered my grief and, as such, have been explored during clinical supervision with Lisa. My triggers include children playing dead, ambulances, Christmas, rainbows, moving between joy and grief, and therapeutic endings. Both clinical supervision and the development of my own internal clinical supervisor have facilitated me to always hold the child's grief at the forefront of my mind, while acknowledging my own grief, and knowing what is *their* personal process and what is *mine*, thus ensuring the safe and ethical practice of play therapy. All the vignettes have been anonymised to protect the identity of the children and families I have worked with.

## Playing "dead" and falling asleep in sessions

Revi is a five-year-old boy whose maternal aunt died. His aunt had played a significant role in his early years, providing childcare when his parents were at work. Revi was referred for play therapy as his school had expressed concerns to his mother about some behavioural changes, including destructive behaviour, demanding high levels of attention from teaching staff and difficulty socialising with his peers. Revi's mother had also become concerned about his behaviour at home. She reported he would shout at anyone who mentioned his aunt's name and then would run away to his room. During the systemic intake process, including an assessment with Revi's mother, I learned that Revi had not been told of his aunt's palliative diagnosis and nor did he attend the funeral as it was perceived he was too young. Furthermore, there had been additional secondary losses following the aunt's death, including family relationship breakdown, arguments and the death of Revi's pet. The family appeared to find it hard to communicate in an open and age-appropriate way. Nevertheless, with the support of school, they were able to identify his struggle and seek bereavement support and guidance (Mallon, 2018; Rolls, 2004; Silverman, 2000). In clinical supervision, Lisa and I mirrored the importance of honesty when working with bereaved children, by being open and honest about my own experiences and the impact it had on me within the therapeutic relationship. This came more naturally than expected as I had tried to be open and transparent from the moment of Andrew's death. Over the years I have found I am able to have difficult and possibly upsetting conversations with children in an age-appropriate manner. Subsequently, in the first play therapy session with Revi, his aunt's death, and how it made him feel, was named as being a reason for attending sessions (Worden, 1996). This willingness to talk about death and dying as a normal part of life certainly stems from not only my childhood experiences, but also from the way in which I have handled Andrew's death with openness, and at times for me with brutal honesty.

Revi is the child who I probably have been triggered by the most: he looked like Andrew in hair and eye colouring. Towards the end of one session Revi appeared to be "playing dead" and I was profoundly triggered by his play. He had been playing with the doll's house and it had become all of a jumble and everything was turned upside down when he suddenly shut the door of the doll's house and lay on the floor with his legs and arms straight down by his side. He only lay there for a fraction of a second, but it was long enough for me to catch my breath to see he was "playing dead". This was a deep gut-wrenching moment when I remembered

Andrew being laid out, much like in the example I provided earlier. At my next clinical supervision session, I discussed this event with Lisa. We explored the overwhelming feelings Revi had been processing and its impact on me. In a parallel process, I too had had an overwhelming bereavement experience where there had been significant chaos resulting from Andrew's sudden death. Having had this flashback, my autonomic nervous system (ANS) became triggered, and I moved out of "my thinking brain" into a place where I was in a state of alert to the unseen danger, which resulted in a "freeze" response from me (Porges, 2011; Rothschild, 2006). By freezing I was not able to reflect and track Revi's play, as I should have done. Furthermore, as the end of the session approached, instead of bringing it to an end therapeutically, I allowed the play to continue for a few minutes longer, permitting Revi to move out of the "playing dead" phase and return to playing with the doll's house. This experience and my response to it may say more about my need to have the chaos resolved and maybe not wanting to have to "tidy it" after he left. There might have been a hope that he sorted out the mess, not leaving me the responsibility of holding his grief as well as my own which was so palpable at the time.

*Having read about the episode of Revi "playing dead" in Sarah's process notes, I asked to see it for myself on her video. It turned out to be so fleeting – as she concedes earlier, possibly even less than a second – that it would have passed me by entirely had Revi been my client. It may or may not have been significant to Revi himself and perhaps held little conscious or unconscious meaning to him, but the fact that it made such a big impact on Sarah was what I needed to address in supervision. As clinical supervisors we need to be alert to both sides of the parallel processes in front of us, and to periodically redirect our focus onto the needs of our supervisees, thereby improving the efficacy of their practice with their young clients and enhancing their availability to meet the children's needs.*

This vignette illustrates how hard it can be to bear witness to children's suffering, showing understanding and acceptance, all the while remaining congruent (Landreth, 2012). At times during play therapy, I can become sleepy, my mind can wander and I can find it difficult to focus on the child and the child's play. These somatic responses were explored in clinical supervision. Lisa wondered if at these times I was trying to self-soothe by becoming disconnected from the pain the child was experiencing, how it was triggering my own pain, and becoming emotionally overwhelmed (Fig. 4.1), to the point of moving into a fight, flight or freeze response (Porges, 2011). Siegel's (1999) *Window of Tolerance* has been a useful model to help me understand more about these auto-responses and how our arousal states are affected by our experiences. Lisa and I discussed ways of grounding myself before, during and after therapeutic sessions to reduce the impact of these somatic experiences (Rothschild, 2006). This included laying my hands in the sand tray prior to seeing a child, holding the hem of my top to stay grounded, and post sessions doing body brushing and maintaining process notes all in order to stay with the child's process congruently and to remain within my own window of tolerance (Siegel, 1999). I was always conscious that "the ability

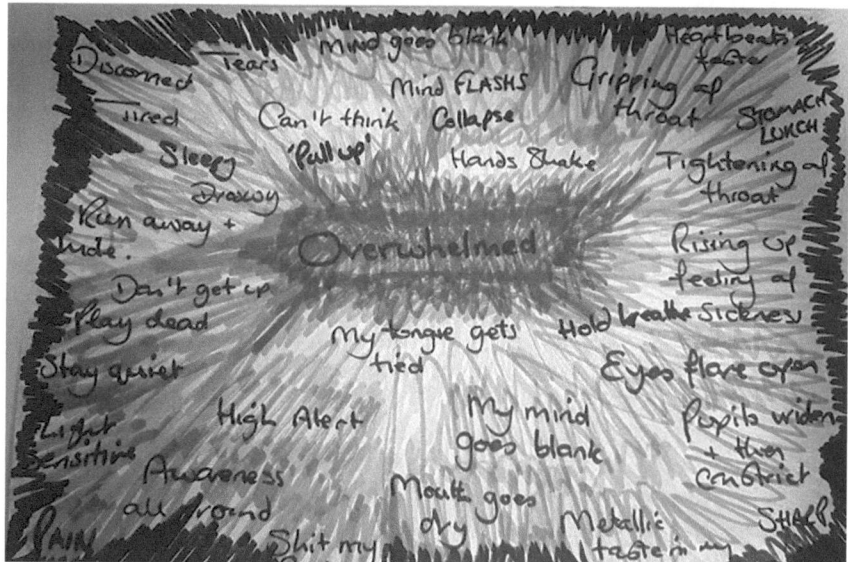

*Figure 4.1* Picture of being overwhelmed

to release background noise and thoughts so that pure contact can take place is a skill of focus or mindfulness that benefits play therapy practice" (Ray, 2011: 75).

## Running away hard from ambulances

Iris attended play therapy when she was 11 years old. Her grandfather had died when she was eight years old. Amongst her mother's concerns was that Iris was having frequent nightmares causing her to be excessively tired in school and struggling to concentrate. Iris was a cognitively able child and she was able to verbalise many of her difficult thoughts and feelings. In one session Iris told me about how whenever she saw ambulances it upset her, and she did not like ambulances, as she still remembered when her grandfather was taken to hospital for the last time by ambulance. While she told this story, I was not aware of my own unconscious processes and leapt from being non-directive to giving her advice and information on how she can help soothe herself when she sees ambulances. It was only in clinical supervision a few days later that I realised I too am triggered by ambulances as one was called when Andrew died. This was followed by a harrowing journey to the hospital as I held Andrew, dead in my arms, all the way to Accident and Emergency. In my need to move away from my own grief and trauma, instead of empathically responding to Iris's struggle and being child-led, I jumped into solving the problem for Iris by becoming more directive in providing cognitive behavioural solutions to this emotional difficulty.

*Occasionally I perceived that Sarah had a tendency to revert to her familiar social worker habits and to become more psychoeducational than therapeutic in her responses. This is characteristic of many students who have to unlearn old professional techniques before consolidating new ones, but it is striking that it occurred most obviously for Sarah when it coincided with a personal trigger to which she reacted defensively. This self-protective response of avoiding emotion in favour of intellectual instruction/didacticism, or of leaping into problem-solving mode, was one she was able to acknowledge readily and thus redress in future.*

*On reflection, as we have worked on this chapter together, it has struck me that Sarah's occasional regression to psychoeducational mode stemmed from moments when her well-developed Rogerian attitude of empathy, essential for all play therapists, spilled over into "overidentification". The enhanced empathy that came from her own experience of bereavement could be viewed as a positive, but equally erosion of the essential "as if" quality of empathy could have led her to make assumptions that were more about her own experiences than that of the child, and/or lead her to self-defensive strategies as she describes above with Iris. She was very conscious of this risk of overidentifying and has said she would not, for example, take on a case of a cot death. In this context, we talked together about the poignant metaphor of the parallel sets of footprints in the sand: the play therapist's role is to walk alongside the child in the journey, but not to step exactly into their footprints so they become blurred into one – nor to "carry" the child so that again there is only one set of prints. We later extended this metaphor and pondered on the presence of a third set of footprints in the sand: mine walking alongside hers. Keeping those footprints clearly distinguishable, and moving forward positively in parallel, became another supervisory task, but one that I have perhaps only appreciated in hindsight.*

## Christmas – "tackling the turkey in the room"

Christmas is an annual event. There is no escaping it, as Christmas is present in my life on a daily basis, as well as being played out in the play therapy room. For many, Christmas is a time for celebration and being together with family. However, for those who are bereaved, it can be an exceedingly difficult time as the separation from one's loved one becomes even more poignant and painful. For me though, it is also the anniversary of Andrew's death. Over time I have become adept at navigating Christmas and the highs and lows it brings me, but it is not without its challenges, and every year is different. I find Christmassy smells, decorations and festivities – all triggers of deep personal trauma. Initially, when I joined the hospice, I tried to "soldier on" through the Christmas and New Year week but I have learned I need to take time off at Christmas, stepping back from therapeutic work for my own well-being. Certainly, when I first began working in the hospice, I found it difficult to manage people's good wishes for a lovely Christmas, but I have learned to grin and bear it, and to know that these wishes are given with good intentions. I know children are trying to navigate the same journey I have made in trying to make sense of the festive season while also experiencing feelings of loss (Mallon, 2018). In bereavement, children and adults can experience guilt and shame for being happy, continuing to be alive and living their lives (Di Ciacco, 2008; Harris, 2020; Stroebe & Schut, 1999; Worden, 1996). My own personal process and developed understanding of these bereavement experiences have enabled me to therapeutically hold and be with the child's process.

*As we approached the first Christmas break of the supervisory relationship, we explored together the language used to explain to clients, and their families, that Sarah would be taking more time off work than the norm. As mentioned earlier, the importance of self-care was regularly underscored, and in fact occasionally I took a leaf out of her book as I concede this is one of the aspects of my own practice that I do not always pay enough respect to. This touches upon my learning from Sarah, which is another aspect of our shared experience worth reflecting briefly upon: that is that supervision can be, indeed should be, a two-way or mutual learning experience. More than once she subtly reminded me to prioritise my own well-being and personal needs, a key example being when my mother suddenly died, towards the end of Sarah's training. Her empathic awareness of my need to take time out to grieve in the immediate aftermath of my own loss exemplified the reciprocal nature of our relationship. This was a poignant example of when having a supervisee who is an expert in dealing with bereavement issues was an unexpected bonus!*

## Sunshine and showers make rainbows

Kiran was five-years-old when he came to me for play therapy. His maternal grandfather had died when Kiran was four. He played a significant caring role in Kiran's life as the family all lived together in a multi-generational household. Kiran's mother, a single mother, was concerned that since starting school Kiran had become clingier, especially to her, and having been dry at night he was suddenly bed-wetting. When Kiran started play therapy, he did not want the play therapy room door to be shut and he asked to see his mother, who was sitting in the waiting room. Kiran would nip out to see she was there and run back into the playroom. The first thing Kiran did in the playroom was to paint a rainbow and throughout his therapeutic sessions, he painted and drew rainbows. Initially, these were rainbows that became muddy brown puddles with large swathes of black paint across the paper. These pictures were so laden with paint that I had to place another piece of paper underneath in order to lift it off the table: this was indeed a "heavy" rainbow to carry, metaphorically and literally, maybe for both of us (Goodyear-Brown, 2019; Mills & Crowley, 2014). As the therapeutic relationship developed, I became aware of Kiran's deep need for making sense of his loss through the metaphor of a rainbow. The brown, muddy pictures became lighter and brighter in both colour and paint. Eventually, I sensed he was getting ready for the sessions to come to an end when his rainbows were drawn using colouring pencils with just a line or two of black amongst the other colours.

In clinical supervision, I have been able to explore the metaphor of rainbows within children's play, and how it triggers my own grief at a somatic level. Whenever I see rainbows, whether in or out of the therapeutic relationship, I physically experience catching my breath and my chest tightens, for at Andrew's funeral *Somewhere Over the Rainbow* was played. During my journey as a bereaved play therapist, I have seen the symbolism of the rainbow holding deep significance not just for myself but also for the children I work with. Rainbows are created by simultaneous sunshine and showers, correlating to joy and sadness, both found in grief. Rainbows are in essence a symbol of hope, as mythology promises that at the end of each rainbow there is the hope of a pot of gold (Chevalier & Gheerbrant, 1996). Rainbows are created by the refraction of sunlight through the raindrops, just as in bereavement there can be healing through the congruent grieving process where both grief and joy come together. Stroebe and Schut's (1999) *Dual Process Model* of the need for movement between *grief-oriented* and *restoration-oriented loss* for the development of resilience is reflected in the term "Puddle Jumping" (Crossley & Sheppard, 2001). Bereaved children are described as jumping in and out of their grief as they feel psychologically able. By creating the artwork of rainbows there is the possibility for the projection of *Self* and in becoming able to understand one's experience of grief and joy (Mills & Crowley, 2014).

*An essential part of the clinical supervision process was Sarah's ability to discuss her response to rainbows and how they triggered her own personal process. With greater self-awareness, she later told me that instead of catching her breath, and her ANS being activated, she could internally smile to herself, consciously just acknowledging the profound symbolic significance of rainbows for her, and quite possibly for the child as well (Rothschild, 2006).*

## Finding joy when bereaved

When Phoenix was eight-years-old, her father died. She was referred as her mother was concerned she was struggling with her loss. She did not play with other children as much as she used to. School also commented Phoenix was finding it difficult to concentrate and they would often find her daydreaming. Throughout most of her time in play therapy, she played a single card game. In the early sessions, Phoenix expressed high levels of need to control the game by creating her own rules in order for her to win the game. In the therapy playroom, where there is permissiveness, children can externalise control, find their balance and develop abilities to exercise internal control (Rotter, 1954). This was true for Phoenix, as sessions went on and the card game continued, she was eventually able to play using the stated rules of the game. Phoenix moved from exhibiting the smallest of reactions to losing or winning, to being able to truly experience the highs and lows of the game. In one session I was rather enjoying the game and almost forgot I was the play therapist. I relished the fact I had been able to celebrate winning when I was suddenly overcome with guilt. I discussed these feelings in clinical supervision. Lisa and I explored how feelings of guilt and shame can be triggered when, as a bereaved person, one is feeling happy. Tonkin's (1996) model of *Growing Around the Grief* illustrates how over time one's grief, as one's love, for the significant person remains the same size, but *one* has grown bigger around the grief. In this growth there is the potential to hold both the grief and the joy at the same time, which is an essential component of the grieving process, much like the analogy of rainbows needing both sunshine and showers. Through the process of clinical supervision, I was able to reflect on my own feelings of guilt and shame, and how at times I felt guilt over feeling happiness after Andrew's death. This insight into my own personal process helped me to have a deeper understanding of Phoenix's own experience of grieving as she too struggled in moving between grief and joy.

*In Sarah's notes on later sessions with Phoenix, which coincided with the anniversary of her father's death, Sarah indicated her own physical pain and tiredness and her anxiety about how the sessions would go. We discussed in supervision the parallels between her own physical disabilities and those children and families affected by a life-limiting illness. Several times her reflections were about feeling "overwhelmed" (even " . . . by work, life and the universe"!) yet towards the end of her work with Phoenix, she experienced fun and connection. This led to an important discussion about the guilt Sarah felt at feeling so relaxed with Phoenix and she made the insightful link to the release of tension she had felt when watching "Mamma Mia" on New Year's Eve just a week after Andrew's death and being able to laugh. She recalled this had given her hope that she could/would survive. Together we considered the therapeutic value of having pure fun with a child – they can be sad but allowed to feel happy too: the sunshine and the showers can co-exist.*

## Saying goodbye to children

As each child leaves, I know I have learned from them. I know I will hold a bit of them in my heart. I hope as they wave goodbye that I have been a good *Helper* in their *Hero's Journey*. I will always feel a sense of sadness when I say goodbye to a client, which reminds me of and resonates at a deep level with my final goodbye to Andrew. However, there is always the knowledge that they go on, as I bid them farewell. I have a greater sense of hope and satisfaction when the end of the therapeutic journey has come. In the bereavement service where I work, play therapy sessions are provided in an initial block of 12 sessions with the option of providing more sessions if needed. Knowing where a child is in the play therapy process is an essential therapeutic skill and the planning of the end of therapy starts at the beginning of the therapeutic journey (Yasenik & Gardner, 2012). Landreth (2012: 349) also identifies "the ending of the therapeutic relationship . . . is just as important as the beginning of the relationship and should be dealt with openly". In a bereavement service, "endings", and how they are achieved therapeutically, are even more crucial as they resonate with the child's own experience of endings, that is the death of someone significant (Worden, 1996). However, knowing how to end interventions has evolved over time. Initially when discussing endings with Lisa I wanted a celebration. This might have reflected my own need and desire for endings to be happy, avoiding the child's feelings of sadness, and experiencing another relationship ending. Klass et al. (1996) argue the need for those bereaved to maintain a connection with their loved one by having *Continuing Bonds*. These bonds need attention and tending to, through continually holding the significant person who died in mind, through both inner and outer expressions of memorial. Therefore, it is imperative the therapeutic journey mirrors healthy endings and the maintaining of *Continuing Bonds* as well. In clinical supervision I learned about having *Farewell Feasts* and being able to acknowledge both the sadness and the joy about sessions ending. I also developed a "VIP" ticket that children could give to their parent/carer after they left, to be able to come and visit the hospice and myself if the need arose. Thus, enabling children to know that both the hospice and I go on, and they can have a lifetime connection with the hospice if they so wish, and ensuring the underlying message that they too can have a *Continuing Bond* with their loved one forever.

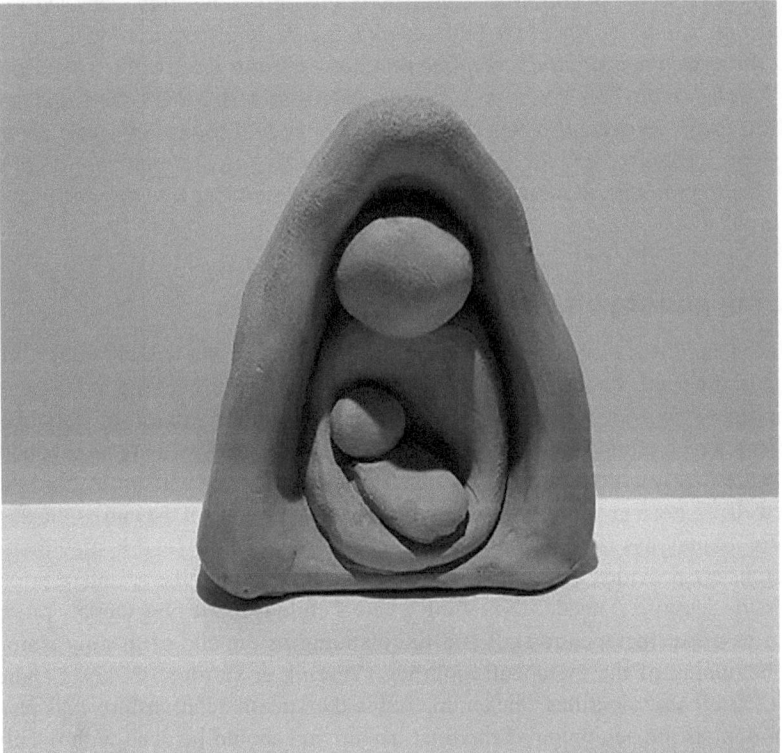

*Figure 4.2* Sculpture of the held mother holding a child

I have reflected that with each goodbye to a child, I feel a sense of loss which is rooted in my loss of Andrew which is a loss I need to resolve myself. Initially, this was solely through clinical supervision but as I have grown in skill and confidence my own "internal supervisor" has grown (Gordon Clark, 2019; McCann, 2017). After one such ending session with a child, I needed to process the sadness I felt in saying goodbye to this child and to acknowledge how underlying that loss was of course the loss of Andrew. I decided to externalise that loss in clay (see Fig. 4.2). This embodied processing resulted in my own internal supervisor being activated, allowing me the time to sit with the loss of another child while also recognising the hope that came with this therapeutic ending. In this piece of self-reflection, I find myself holding the symbolic child, client and Andrew, while being held myself. As a practising Christian, the "holding" of me was that of God, but maybe it is also being held in mind by my supervisor simultaneously. Maybe in retrospect this piece also reflects something of the supervisor/supervisee relationship because the mother/therapist holding the child is also being held too, resonating with the footprints in the sand metaphor used earlier.

## Not letting go but moving forward

As I approached the end of my year as a newly qualified play therapist, Lisa and I agreed that we would bring our clinical supervision relationship to an end. It was not that I no longer needed supervision, rather that I wanted to move on to another clinical supervisor who lived closer to me. The changing dynamic between us also enabled us to shift the balance in our relationship from being supervisee/ supervisor to one of being peers and co-authors for this chapter. Having made this decision, it gave us the golden opportunity to model good practice by processing the journey we had been on together in clinical supervision. I created a sand tray of my journey with Lisa, as my *Helper*, in our final session (see Fig. 4.3). This sand tray included all my play therapy clients represented in miniature form. The sand tray begins with Andrew's coffin, with my husband standing, ever supportive, behind me, then winds backwards and forwards from right to left, through each therapeutic experience, every child I worked with and the obstacles and hurdles I have had to overcome. In the latter half of the sand tray, the wooden egg represents finding a new life as a play therapist, the wooden coffin had been transformed into a life affirming egg.

*The creation and shared contemplation of this final sand tray was a deeply moving experience for us both. One of the miniatures is a red motorbike, which I gave Sarah as a transitional object (Winnicott, 1971), representing the symbolic continuing bond between us, and as a metaphor for the next stage of our relationship: I was confident that the momentum was enough for me to let go and that she would keep her balance going forward, if she watched out for potholes and remembered to keep enough fuel in her tank. She was ready to journey on without me (Klass et al., 1996).*

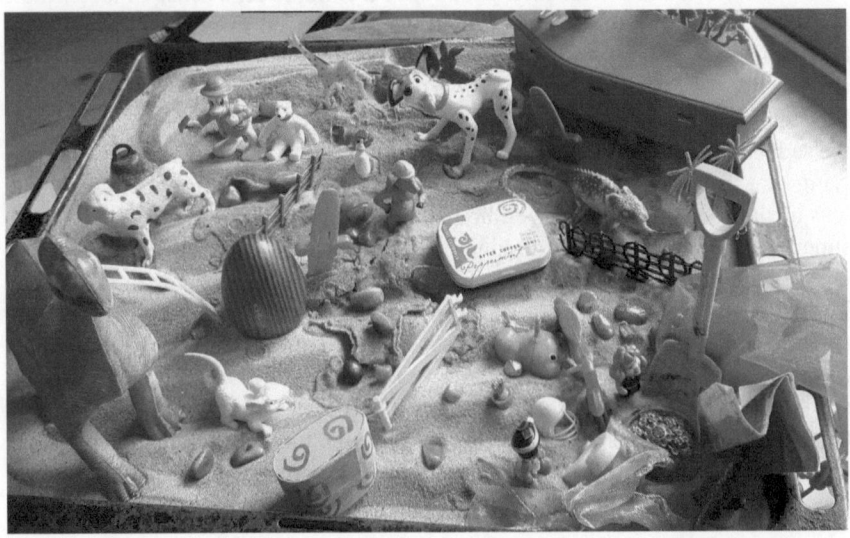

*Figure 4.3* Ending clinical supervision relationship – sand tray

## Conclusion

The death of Andrew remains a traumatic devastating life event which continues to impact on my life, and I imagine will do so throughout my lifetime. However, through the pain I have found unexpected blessings born out of this unimaginable grief and pain. Paradoxically, his death has been the making of me and led to me becoming a wounded healer. In my woundedness, and with humility and curiosity, I am now able to come alongside other deeply wounded individuals to be *their* helper. It is my experience that clinical supervision and personal therapy, as required by BAPT, have been critical components in this process of coming to this point of healing in my own life – a point of knowing and understanding my *Self*, a process of growth that enabled me to become stronger, more resilient, more hopeful and able to help others. It has been quite a journey, my own *Hero's Journey*, and of finding gold at the end of the rainbow, the gifts from grief and helping others to find their own gifts too.

## References

Axline, V. M. (1969) *Play Therapy*. New York: Ballantine Books (Original work published 1947).

Bercier, M. L. & Maynard, B. R. (2015) Interventions for Secondary Traumatic Stress With Mental Health Workers: A Systematic Review. *Research on Social Work Practice*, 25(1), pp. 81–89.

Bowlby, J. (1973) *Separation: Anxiety & Anger. Attachment and Loss* (vol. 2). London: Hogarth Press.

British Association of Play Therapists. (2021) *Ethical Basis for Good Practice in Play Therapy*. Available at: www.bapt.info/play-therapy/ethical-basis-good-practice-play-therapy/ (Accessed: 28 February 2021).

Campbell, J. (2008) *The Hero With a Thousand Faces* (3rd ed.). Novato, CA: New World Library, The Joseph Campbell Foundation.

Cattanach, A. (2008) *Play Therapy With Abused Children* (2nd ed.). London: Jessica Kingsley Publishers.

Chevalier, J. & Gheerbrant, A. (1996) *Dictionary of Symbols*. London: Penguin Books.

Clarkson, P. (2003) *The Therapeutic Relationship* (2nd ed.). London: Whurr Publishers.

Crossley, D. & Sheppard, K. (2001) *Muddles, Puddles and Sunshine*. Stroud: Hawthorn Press.

Daniels, D. & Jenkins, P. (2010) *Therapy With Children: Children's Rights, Confidentiality, and the Law* (2nd ed.). London: Sage Publications.

Di Ciacco, J. A. (2008) *The Colors of Grief*. Philadelphia: Jessica Kingsley Publishers.

Goodyear-Brown, P. (2019) *Trauma and Play Therapy: Helping Children Heal*. London: Routledge.

Gordon Clark, L. (2019) Training Issues: Before, During and After. In: Ayling, P., Armstrong, H. & Gordon Clark, L. (eds.) *Becoming and Being a Play Therapist: Play Therapy in Practice* (pp. 11–23). London: Routledge.

Harris, S. (2020) Motherhood and the Traumatic Death of One's Child. In: Arnold-Baker, C. (ed.) *The Existential Crisis of Motherhood* (pp. 199–220). London: Palgrave MacMillan.

Hawkins, P. & Shohet, R. (2012) *Supervision in the Helping Professions* (4th ed.). Maidenhead: Open University Press.

Henderson, P., Holloway, J. & Millar, A. (2014) *Practical Supervision: How to Become a Supervisor for the Helping Professions*. London: Jessica Kingsley Publishers.

Hensel, J. M., Ruiz, C., Finney, C. & Dewa, C. S. (2015) Meta-Analysis of Risk Factors for Secondary Traumatic Stress in Therapeutic Work with Trauma Victims. *Journal of Traumatic Stress*, 28(2), pp. 83–91.

Klass, D., Silverman, P. R. & Nickman, S. L. (1996) *Continuing Bonds: An Understanding of Grief*. Washington, DC: Taylor & Francis Publishers.

Lahad, M. (1997) The Story as a Guide to Metaphoric Processes. In: Jennings, S. (ed.) *Dramatherapy: Theory and Practice 3* (vol. 3, pp. 31–42). London: Routledge.

Lahad, M. (2000) *Creative Supervision*. London: Jessica Kingsley Publishers.

Landreth, G. L. (2012) *Play Therapy: The Art of the Relationship* (3rd ed.). London: Routledge.

Le Vay, D. (2016) To Be or Not to Be? The Therapeutic Use of Self Within Child-Centred Play Therapy. In: Le Vay, D. & Cuschieri, E. (eds.) *Challenges in the Theory and Practice of Play Therapy* (pp. 1–17). London: Routledge.

Levine, S. (2005) *Unattended Sorrow: Recovering From Loss and Reviving the Heart*. Emmaus: Rodale.

Luff, J. & Ingham, H. (1955) The Johari Window: A Graphic Model of Interpersonal Awareness. In *Proceedings of the Western Training Laboratory in Group*. Los Angeles: Development UCLA.

Macran, S. & Shapiro, D. (1998) The Role of Personal Therapy for Therapists: A Review. *British Journal of Medical Psychology*, 71, pp. 13–25.

Mallon, B. (2018) *Building Continuing Bonds for Grieving and Bereaved Children*. London: Jessica Kingsley Publishers.

McCann, D. (2017) Supervision: Making It Work for You. In: Bor, R. & Watts, M. (eds.) *The Trainee Handbook: A Guide for Counselling and Psychotherapy Trainees* (4th ed., pp. 346–368). London: Sage Publications.

McCann, J. (2019) The Play Therapist's Personal Therapy. In: Ayling, P., Armstrong, H. & Gordon Clark, L. (eds.) *Becoming and Being a Play Therapist: Play Therapy in Practice* (pp. 24–39). London: Routledge.

McMahon, L. (1992) *The Handbook of Play Therapy*. London: Routledge.

Mills, J. C. & Crowley, R. J. (2014) *Therapeutic Metaphors for Children and the Child Within*. London: Routledge.

Norcross, J. C. & VandenBos, G. R. (2018) *Leaving It at the Office: A Guide to Therapist Self-Care* (2nd ed.). New York: Guilford Press.

Nouwen, H. J. M. (2014) *The Wounded Healer: Ministry in Contemporary Society*. London: Doubleday.

Perry, B. D. (2014) The Cost of Caring: Understanding and Preventing Secondary Traumatic Stress When Working With Traumatized and Maltreated Children. *CTA Parent and Caregiver Education Series*, 2(7). Child Trauma Academy Press. Available at: www.childtrauma.org/trauma-ptsd (Accessed: 14 November 2020).

Platteuw, C. (2019) The Role of Clinical Supervision in Play Therapy Practice. In: Ayling, P., Armstrong, H. & Gordon Clark, L. (eds.) *Becoming and Being a Play Therapist: Play Therapy in Practice* (pp. 40–54). London: Routledge.

Porges, S. W. (2011) *The Polyvagal Theory: Neurophysiological Foundations of Emotions, Attachment, Communication, Self-regulation*. London: W. W. Norton & Company.

Ray, D. (2011) *Advanced Play Therapy: Essential Conditions, Knowledge, and Skills for Child Practice*. London: Routledge.

Rogers, C. R. (1957) The Necessary and Sufficient Conditions of Therapeutic Personality Change. *Journal of Consulting Psychology*, 21(1), pp. 95–103. (Reprint).

Rolls, L. (2004) Families and Children Facing Loss and Bereavement. In: Payne, S., Seymour, S. & Ingleton, C. (eds.) *Palliative Care Nursing: Principles and Evidence for Practice* (pp. 555–576). Maidenhead: Open University Press.

Rose, C. (2012) Self-Awareness in Psychotherapy and Counselling. In: Rose, C. (ed.) *Self-Awareness and Personal Development: Resources for Psychotherapists and Counsellors* (pp. 1–13). Basingstoke: Palgrave Macmillan.

Rosenberg, K. (2015) Finding the Gifts in Grief. *Bereavement Care*, 34(2), pp. 40–42.

Rothschild, B. (2006) *Help for the Helper: The Psychophysiology of Compassion Fatigue and Vicarious Trauma*. London: Norton Professional Books.

Rotter, J. B. (1954) *Social Learning and Clinical Psychology*. New York: Prentice-Hall.

Ryan, V. & Wilson, K. (2000) *Case Studies in Non-Directive Play Therapy* (2nd ed.). London: Jessica Kingsley Publishers.

Sawyer, G. (2015) Self-Care in Hospice Work. *Therapy Today*, 7, pp. 22–25.

Siegel, D. (1999) *The Developing Mind: How Relationships and the Brain Interact to Shape Who We Are*. New York: Guilford Press.

Silverman, P. R. (2000) *Never Too Young to Know: Death in Children's Lives*. Oxford: Oxford University Press.

Stoltenberg, C. D. & McNeill, B. W. (2010) *IDM Supervision: An Integrative Developmental Model for Supervising Counselors and Therapists* (3rd ed.). New York: Routledge.

Stone, C. (2019) Bereavement, Loss, and Play Therapy. In: Ayling, P., Armstrong, H. & Gordon Clark, L. (eds.) *Becoming and Being a Play Therapist: Play Therapy in Practice* (pp. 201 211). London: Routledge.

Stroebe, M. & Schut, H. (1999) The Dual Process Model of Coping With Bereavement: Rationale and Description. *Death Studies*, 23(3), pp. 197–224.

Tonkin, L. (1996) Growing Around Grief – Another Way of Looking at Grief and Recovery. *Bereavement Care*, 15(1), pp. 10–10.

Winnicott, D. W. (1971) *Playing and Reality*. London: Tavistock Publications.

Worden, J. W. (1996) *Children and Grief: When a Parent Dies*. New York: The Guilford Press.

Worden, J. W. (2003) *Grief Counselling and Grief Therapy: A Handbook for the Mental Health Practitioner* (3rd ed.). London: Routledge.

Yasenik, L. & Gardner, K. (2012) *Play Therapy Dimensions Model*. London: Jessica Kingsley Publishers.

# Chapter 5

# Shame

## Healing and beyond

*Francesca Wright*

## Part 1

*There once was a house on the top of a tall hill. It was not like the other houses nearby. Dark clouds gathered over it, and thunder raged as lightning struck out at its chimney tops. Nobody visited the house. Nobody wanted to know what was inside.*

*Inside the house lived a boy and his mother. He was just a little boy and the stormy house had often made him feel scared. The little boy saw the most terrifying shadows. They reminded him of the scariest of storms. He could often be found making a storm of his own in the nearby forest. The little boy's mother tried so many things to make the shadows leave, but nothing seemed to work. She worried that the shadows would live in the walls forever.*

During my final year of the Play Therapy MA at the University of Roehampton, I completed my dissertation, a heuristic enquiry seeking to understand the phenomenon of shame, its manifestation during play therapy training and the potential for such training to aid healing. Three years later, I am revisiting my training experience and hope to illuminate further on the process and what play therapists can learn from their own shame. In this chapter, I have included extracts from my own journals and work during my training, anonymised vignettes of student and clinical practice and some of my own reflections.

Shame is a complex emotion. It is profoundly personal and manifests in unique and nuanced ways. Re-examining my time in training has been painful. Ironically, within my own research, I managed to keep much of myself and my own shame under wraps. This chapter provides opportunity to explore a more personal account of shame, but to expose my own process is challenging and, paradoxically, I worry it is self-indulgent somehow. I may start with a caveat; I am no expert on shame. I am still coming to terms with its elements even now. But perhaps I can share something of what I learnt during my training and in the years that followed.

True to its surreptitious nature, literature on shame is limited, often focusing on client shame as opposed to exploring therapists' personal shame. The linguistic roots of the word "shame" highlight something of its nature as it is derived from

DOI: 10.4324/9781003017271-5

the Germanic word "skem/skam" (Wurmser, 1981). The etymology of this is the Indo-European word "kami/kem" meaning, "to cover, to veil, to hide" with the "s" prefix adding reflexive meaning "to cover oneself" (Wurmser, 1981: 29). This emphasises "hiding" as a fundamental part of shame.

Given shame's ability to lurk hidden and undetected, finding an all-encompassing definition is elusive. We often struggle to distinguish shame from other painful emotions such as guilt or embarrassment which further complicates our understanding of it. The terms shame, guilt, embarrassment and humiliation are used interchangeably and perhaps, catachrestically. Feelings of shame arise due to the emphasis placed on the self, rather than the behaviour (Lewis, 1971; Brown, 2007). The distinction lies between feeling you have *done* something bad and feeling that you *are* inherently bad. Brown conceptualised her own definition of shame as "the intensely painful feeling or experience of believing we are flawed and therefore unworthy of acceptance and belonging" (2007: 5).

## Shame in literature

Within early psychoanalysis, shame was substantially overlooked, in comparison to emotions like guilt. This may have laid the foundations for a wider avoidance throughout history as the first, and most in-depth exploration of shame, came from Helen Block Lewis in 1971, who compiled clinical material into her book *Shame and Guilt in Neurosis*. Block Lewis (1971) highlighted shame as "contagious" and identified its propensity towards remaining concealed, which encourages others, like the therapist, to hide from it too. Lewis identified previously unrecognised distinctions between shame and guilt, helping to distinguish shame as an emotion in its own right.

Shame has detrimental, long-term impacts on an individual's functioning and development. Links have been made between shame and wide-ranging problems, including substance and alcohol abuse (Dearing et al., 2005), psychological difficulties such as depression and anxiety (Shahar et al., 2015; Hedman et al., 2013), and risk-taking behaviours (Stuewig et al., 2015). Research has also highlighted that shame may also be experienced more intensely by those who have endured adverse childhood experiences, such as abuse and maltreatment (Andrews & Hunter, 1997; Webb et al., 2007; Shahar et al., 2015). Given these complex origins and potentially harmful consequences, shame is clearly worthy of greater understanding.

Shame is a natural emotional response, experienced by us all, appearing early in the life of a developing child, somewhere between 14 and 16 months (Schore, 1991, 1994). With new developments in neuroscience, we understand a great deal more about how important our early years are in creating the foundations that shape us. Our brains, specifically the pre-frontal cortex, which helps in regulating emotions, develop further in response to positive social interactions (Gerhardt, 2004). As infants grow, their burgeoning sense of autonomy and new-found independence can increase the potential for them to enter into danger. A parent's stern response forces the child to stop what they are doing, which can induce shame. Badenoch (2008) suggests that parents who respond empathically to children can effectively repair these ruptures in synchronicity. A punitive or indifferent parent may not respond quickly or adequately enough, so children learn to expect anger and rejection. Furthermore, Badenoch (2008) highlights that the latter parenting styles mean "shame-prone" persons regard themselves as defective, unworthy and likely to be rejected, because of ingrained "cortical" representations.

Whilst continual exposure to shame is detrimental to overall functioning and brain development, there are conflicting arguments as to whether shame serves positive functions. Like guilt, shame has been argued to be a sufficient motivational factor towards change. Individuals may examine and alter their functioning as it often results in denunciation of the "self" if a person's behaviour is identified as an infraction of a societal or moral code (Epstein & Falconier, 2011). However, whilst guilt drives us towards repair, shame can also be experienced as a shutting down and avoidance to rebuke negative feelings (Greenberg & Iwakabe, 2011).

Rogers suggested that the therapist's capacity to facilitate development and change in a client is "a measure of the growth I have achieved in myself" (1967: 56). The therapist's emotional maturity and growth is a necessary ingredient in their client work. Shame can have destructive consequences however, impacting on an individual's capacity to empathise because shame redirects focus onto the self, as opposed to others (Brown, 2007; Tangney & Dearing, 2002).

## Shame and therapeutic training models

Shame is a rarely covered subject in therapeutic training courses with many therapists having not studied it at all (Brown et al., 2011). With training courses often taught in line with a therapeutic model, decisions are made about which subjects are most valuable. Cultural expectations and norms likely influence "acceptable" topics. When we do not address difficult issues, we contribute to furthering the mystery and shame around them. Training programmes may collude in topics remaining "taboo". In play therapy, we provide children with a space to fully express and explore their feelings and yet, our training environments may inadvertently heighten feelings of shame and cause students to minimise or shield others from their challenges and difficulties.

Higher education institutes face a balancing act between ensuring academic success is facilitated whilst also encouraging both emotional development and managing student well-being. For the student, there is also a need to protect oneself and defend your right to be on a training course in the first place. As suggested by Adams, "Stirring up the mud underneath is just a little too unsettling for most of us, exposing as it does the less noble side of ourselves". (2014: 14). Despite best efforts to create an environment of sharing, openness and vulnerability, there is an underlying expectation that you will remain mentally well during training. Students' own desire for professional development and academic success may result in reluctance in sharing, and the environment might restrict trainees' ability to be congruent about its impact on them. Furthermore, we all have different tolerance levels for disclosure and a very real fear of jeopardising one's position on your course can exist.

There is undoubtedly a cultural perception of therapists as omnibenevolent beings as opposed to human beings with faults and difficulties of their own. Idealised identities can contribute to feelings of shame, fear and disconnection (Brown, 2007). There can be significant personal conflict in managing a high-pressured academic environment, alongside ideals about therapists. Therapists have a duty and are expected to have "worked through" their own material and I often felt unable to meet these standards. My core belief as a shame-prone person was that I was "defective" or "bad".

## Part 2

*One day, the boy's mother heard a small voice. "My name is Spider. I've been sent to help", said a spider from the window. The spider listened as the mother told her all about the scary storms and the shadows. She told the spider that when the storms had been at their worst, she and the little boy had not come out of the house, as the house locked itself up tight so no one could escape. The spider explained that when things have been stormy, it can be helpful to go on a special journey to help children make sense of things.*

## Why play therapy?

I began my career working with children and young people affected by serious crimes. I became increasingly frustrated with the levels of support I was able to provide and I was often a holding space for those who desperately needed therapeutic support but would probably never get it. There was only so far I could go with them. My need to help others intensified and my decision to train as a play therapist was cemented. Despite feeling I had overcome great personal and professional challenges; I was still unprepared for the turmoil the training unearthed.

As I navigated the new world of play therapy training and learnt about the impact certain experiences can have on children, I had trouble making sense of my own childhood and the decisions that were made around my care. My own childhood was not always happy. I was the only child of a single mother. My father had been absent as he struggled with drug addiction, being in and out of prison and serious mental health problems. Between the ages of four and 12, I saw him twice. My mother worked full-time meaning much of my day-to-day care was left to my maternal Aunt, where I often felt I was unwanted and an outsider.

Shame surfaced during my training as I questioned how I could heal others, whilst feeling overwhelmed by own my "wounds". Many of those who are attracted to psychotherapy and counselling identify as having experienced "personal wounding" with abuse, childhood and poor mental health being the most common (Barr, 2006). Whilst there is no definitive list of what causes shame, there are often common categories such as family, trauma and appearance (Brown, 2012). Carl Jung proposed that "the doctor is effective only when he himself is affected. Only the wounded physician heals" (1963: 133). The therapist's own experience of psychological distress is suggested as a necessary ingredient for therapy to be of value to a client. Inspired by Chiron, a centaur in Greek mythology, with an incurable wound, the term is applied to those in helping professions with the belief that through their own wounded afflictions, they can heal others. For some, like me, the "re-opening" of personal wounds and increased mental vulnerability may exacerbate shame.

## Towards healing

I was 25 when I started training and had many hopes for the experience to come. Naively, I felt I had dealt with many of my "issues". I had already been in therapy twice before and felt I had completed a significant portion of my "personal growth". How wrong I was. Instead, I became introverted, withdrawn and reclusive. I worried constantly but was determined to "keep it all together". Parallel to this, my friends were establishing themselves in careers, buying properties, getting engaged. I felt I was going backwards. In some respects, I was revisiting experiences I had long since buried. My confidence and self-esteem fell to an all-time low and I felt trapped in a relationship I could not seem to escape.

## Part 3

*The spider spun a long string of silk around the boy. His whole body started spinning very fast and he felt a little nervous. What if she was not a nice spider after all? The silk unravelled and the little boy was surprised to see they were not in the attic anymore, but in the middle of a forest. The little boy marvelled at all the things there were to do and together they played many things.*

## Supervision

The fear of exposure is very real for shame-prone people. Shame causes us to retreat and inhibits us from sharing our stories. I was adept at hiding and unable to validate my own feelings and experiences. Shame-prone individuals are accustomed to censoring ourselves, and our shame can lead us to remain quiet, which may increase our struggles within the supervision setting. Non-disclosure in therapists often relates to feeling information is unimportant or too personal (Ladany et al., 1996). Given shame's furtive nature, and its limited focus within training settings, students may not have the necessary understanding to identify it. When we self-censor personal issues triggered in client sessions, we can be further vulnerable as we grapple with our own and potential client shame too.

*2nd March 2017:*

> *I have been so ill. I have a horrendous cough and a really high temperature. I had pains in my chest from coughing so badly – I was sent home from Uni on Monday. I couldn't sleep and then felt equally awful on Tuesday and left Uni after the lecture. My friend suggested it might be psychosomatic – because of everything I need to get off my chest at the moment.*

Reflection:

> *I am in my first-year placement. I've been battling a few illnesses in a very short space of time and am losing my voice – I worry I will lose it completely – something that has recurred since childhood. Scarlett, a 6-year-old girl I am working with, comes in and immediately sets to work on painting. She is painting a very colourful picture of her mother. She is unusually quiet. Only this painting matters. She grabs a tube of blue glitter and adds some glue to mother's face. She drizzles the glitter in streaks pouring in long lines from her mother's eyes. She tells me "Mummy's crying". I reflect Mummy seems really sad. She tells me, "Mummy's crying because Dean has been bashing her head into the wall".*

Shame can often result in maladaptive behaviours such as avoidance and withdrawal (Nathanson, 1992). My own avoidance meant I struggled to be present with the children I was working with. Any "good" feelings I had about my capacity as a therapist and developing practice were short lived. Supervision reminded me to connect with the feelings and experience of another person, but it was not easy. A therapist's skills lie in their ability to connect meaningfully with another and to function as a vessel for empathy, acceptance and positive regard for a client. Shame can be detrimental for both therapeutic and other relationships (Black et al., 2013). Therapists need to be able to recognise and accurately reflect (at least most of the time) the emotions of others. When we are overwhelmed by our own shame, we are not capable of extending this sort of care to our clients.

However, play therapy provides a unique opportunity to engage in a variety of responsive, supportive relationships and this may facilitate personal growth and development, and counter shame around traumatic experiences. Therapists' own experiences of trauma, whilst receiving clinical supervision, could even result in greater levels of personal growth (Linley & Joseph, 2007). The first people I disclosed the unbridled truth of my relationship to were my supervisor and then my therapist. Up until then, I had only really alluded to some minor issues with a couple of friends who could absolutely see the stress and toll it was taking on me but who I had not felt ready to confide in. Ending this relationship and the child's disclosure on placement all happened in the same week. It took me a long time to be honest about what was happening because of the shame I experienced. I could not possibly have been in a relationship like that. Not after everything I "knew" and all the work I had done around domestic abuse. Having had time to reflect, I see now that there was not just my own shame to deal with during this time.

Supervision may provide a space for exploration of personal experience, which can be a resource rather than a hindrance, with areas seen as "red flags" potentially being beneficial as therapists with similar lived experience to clients may approach issues differently from those without (Timm & Blow, 1999). In the weeks that followed, Scarlett avoided discussing the disclosure, hanging her head when it was mentioned. It transpired that her mother was not happy with her about it. If shame had been a topic we had discussed in more depth within training, there might have been a deeper learning opportunity here for us all, particularly within my supervision group. At the time, I did not have the necessary understanding to truly recognise my own or my client's shame for what it was.

A common theme in my own research was that myself and my co-researchers had all experienced significant or repeated traumatic losses. All of us seemed to have internalised these traumas as being a direct result of something "bad" within us or something "missing". Shame transforms loss and trauma into perceived deficits. As highlighted by Miller, cultural expectations often force us, "not to take one's own suffering seriously" (1990: 5). Shame prevents us from acknowledging our experiences, empathising with ourselves and expressing our feelings. Shame draws us inwards and towards the "self", causing us to question our worth. Internalised shame functions as "the dark mirror within" (Gilbert, 2011: 328), reflecting back to us an image of ourselves as not being "enough". Shame convinces us that we are deserving of these "bad" experiences, somehow to blame, or lacking.

Supervision can provide an opportunity for shame to be worked through (Ladany et al., 2011; Hahn, 2001). But that would require supervisors or supervisees to be able to recognise shame lurking and to bring it into discussion. If we are not trained with a goal to understanding shame and recognising it, how can we possibly identify it when it surfaces? Despite the best intentions to emulate the principles we adopt as play therapists within our supervisory environments, the trainee's lack of experience creates an inevitable power imbalance. As such, supervision within appraising and performance-based environments such as higher education settings has the potential to be a breeding ground for shame.

To risk putting yourself "out there" to be "critiqued", even by the most sensitive of supervisors, feels overwhelmingly threatening. We often measure ourselves and our lives against unrealistic and impossible "idealised" images. Our drive towards unrealistic perfection causes shame when we cannot match up to this "ideal" self. Supervisors can support therapists to set aside idealistic, perfectionist standards and encourage self-compassion, enabling shame to become an opportunity for personal growth (Sanftner & Tantillo, 2011). Shame is complex, layered and reinforced by internalised societal pressures and expectations. Shame tells us that we are never enough, have enough or do enough. I not only learnt a lot from my supervision group but also experienced chronic levels of anxiety that contributed to avoidance. Individual supervision provided a gentler, less threatening environment and stopped me from evaluating myself against others. For some of us, we must feel safe before we can be challenged or pushed further.

Like the children we work with, we bring with us whole histories that have influenced our expectations and perceptions of ourselves – our schooling, parental expectations, cultural influence and more. Shame creates fear that our "flaws" will be laid bare in front of others, causing them to judge and reject us. For some of us, just being "seen" by others is painful.

*I am working with Chloe, an 8-year-old girl who may be here because of human trafficking and it is hoped she will shortly be adopted. She often stares at me and then seemingly becomes overwhelmed, sometimes hiding or looking at me from behind things. I sense she is at times flooded by the experience of another's gaze. It feels too much. I avert my eyes. She enjoys showing me various gymnastic tricks. But despite enjoying the presence of another, she has a low level of tolerance for it. She must get everything right. There is no room for error. She becomes frustrated with herself over small mistakes. Sometimes she stands frozen, looking uncertain, uncomfortable. I reflect that she does not always like it when I watch. One day, she asks me to turn away. She is practising things before she shows me. Wanting to get it just right before she lets me see, hoping that if I do not see the "mistakes" she will not be rejected.*

## Experiential process group

Despite shame's connections to intersubjective experience and relationships, it contributes to feelings of "otherness" and separation, impacting our capacity for relationships (Tangney & Dearing, 2002). This sensation of being the "other", lonely and isolated, which accompanies shame, further emphasises our feelings of being unworthy. We experience ourselves as not belonging.

*22nd February 2017*

> *I feel emotionally the course has been very demanding . . . I can't find my words or ability to be honest about what I am thinking or feeling. The course has made me so introverted. I feel I don't know who I am anymore. I felt angry in Process Group and full of rage. I don't know why it makes me feel so angry but it does.*

During training, we are not just individuals but also members of a group. For some, this brings comfort, for those like me, it increases risk and fear of exposure. The presence of others, feelings of self-consciousness, the stimulation of regressive desires and inevitable comparison in group settings can heighten shame (Gans & Weber, 2000). Much literature exists to support group therapy settings as helpful in combatting feelings of shame (Gans & Weber, 2000; Shapiro & Powers, 2011; Schoenleber & Gratz, 2018). As play therapy students, we do not engage in group therapy as part of training, but the Experiential Process Group and small groups like supervision offer a similar space for reflection and discussion of vulnerabilities and challenges, and may have therapeutic potential.

When I reflect on my own experience of Process Group, and re-read my essays and writing around this time, I am struck by the severity of my feelings, mostly anger and irritation. My lack of contribution and silence became a continual source of frustration. I felt a tension between my resistance of the group and a deep longing to belong. The group can be experienced similarly to that of one's own family (Earley, 2000).

*I never felt I belonged to a "real" family. It was just me and my mother. It was clearly a significant source of stress for my aunt to look after me and her own four children. I dreaded going to her house after school and during the summer holidays. I felt a burning desire to have her attention and recognition, which was nearly always withheld. I was often in "trouble". My cousins would sit excitedly to watch our home videos, whilst I would shrink in horror as we had to relive their finest, and my worst, moments. This included videos where my aunt would shout at me to get out of the way so that she could record her own children and not have me in view. I would memorise the parts where she rejected me so that I could go to the toilet to escape. I did not feel loved, cared about or wanted. The memories that stand out the most are the small actions she took to ensure I remembered I was not her child – not part of her family. Despite being paid by my mother to look after me, which included feeding me, she repeatedly bought her children the exciting muller corner yoghurts and gave me tiny pots. Inevitably, my cousins started to follow suit, often reminding me of my "otherness" – when I'd join in with excitement at my uncle returning home from work, they'd say "that's not your dad. You don't have one".*

My early life experiences of my very first "group" had inevitably shaped my feelings towards and expectations of others. Groups often utilise shame to maintain conformity (Broucek, 1991). Once we understand the transference that can happen within groups, we can see that the feelings "groups" evoke may be related to other experiences. I felt angry when others interrupted the silence, believing it belonged to me. I found group members to be monopolising and this evoked strong feelings of dislike towards them at points. Once I understood this as a possible transference of my feelings towards family members who received attention at my expense, I felt able to connect more openly with others. Acknowledging and accepting these difficult feelings enabled me to form better relationships on the course.

My avoidance has often provided me with safety and allowed me to control my feelings of exposure. Just as our clients have processes for defending themselves, from the child who lashes out at us aggressively to the one who is desperate to build an attachment, therapists and trainees are not immune from their own defensive strategies being played out in training. My own mechanisms make me shut down because I learnt early on that I was not wanted and not "worthy" of being part of a group. Instead, I developed another strategy – if I am going to be a part of a group, then it will be on my own terms.

*14th March 2017*

> *There's a vulnerability attached to sharing in the group space . . . I went in with the expectation that the group would shame and hurt me . . . what is it that makes me hate groups but also want to be a part of one?*

*21st March 2017*

> *During Process Group, there is interest in how poignant and relevant themes coalesce on the course – how familiar feelings are recreated by children we work with. I think about the safeguarding I've had with Scarlett this week. And the fact I finally ended my relationship. My body feels heavy and tight. My heart pounds. Someone mentions the importance of listening to your body – that a painful relationship quite literally gave them a "pain" in the neck and once it ended – the pain was gone. I feel the emotion quite literally bubble out of me and I have to leave. Someone comes to get me. I'm pacing in the toilet – I don't want to go back to the room and face the music. My heart was pumping out of my chest – she said she could hear it! I told them how I had been in a bad relationship and that my mother experienced some similar issues with my father. I told them I hadn't felt able to be part of the group – I hadn't been able to get too close . . . People empathised with me and cried.*

*A few weeks later . . .*

> *"A member of the groups sandtray included a tower – and that represented me. I felt very grateful for that. And accepted. A real acceptance from the group I hadn't felt before. I think ever . . ."*

Process Group has the potential to be a transformative experience during training for those who are shame-prone. Clough (2014) suggests shame signifies the breakdown of relationships and fragmentation of social connections, and that healing transpires when these connections are restored. It is, of course, a risk to speak out and to expose yourself to others. But those who are "shame-resilient" use several strategies to combat shame such as understanding of individual triggers, critical awareness to deconstruct and normalise shame, and the ability to speak out and connect with others (Brown, 2007). Sharing shame is necessary.

## Part 4

*The little boy and the spider travelled through many magical forests together. They played lots and the little boy made many things along the way. After a long journey, the little boy wanted to rest and the spider fashioned a blanket from her silk. The little boy hung it between two large, cotton trees to make a hammock. He climbed inside and the spider gently rocked it. They sat there for some time. Not saying much at all.*

*When he felt strong enough to carry on, the silk unwound and the little boy felt able to stand on his own two feet again. He told the spider he wasn't sure where to go next. But the little boy remembered a slingshot he made earlier. He unwound the silk and told the spider he would use it as a dowsing rod. As they marched onwards, he brushed his hands against the bark of the trees and the petals of the flowers and noticed everything felt more real.*

## Personal therapy

> *Does it hurt?' asked the Rabbit. 'Sometimes', said the Skin Horse, for he was always truthful. 'When you are Real you don't mind being hurt.*
>
> (Williams, 2004)

Trainees are in a unique position, oscillating between many roles – professionals, students, supervisees and therapeutic clients. Personal therapy is an obligatory aspect of many training courses. The value of therapists own personal therapy has been debated for many years, with intermittent research to address its validity. But personal growth is not the central focus of therapeutic training and therapists are ". . . not trained with an overt training goal being to improve their well-being or help them resolve their own identity issues" (McHenry, 1994: 565). Research exploring therapists' views of personal therapy found that many identified both risks and benefits and there are conflicting perspectives of its effectiveness, particularly during training (Macaskill & Macaskill, 1992; McEwan & Duncan, 1993).

I was unprepared for the ferocity and intensity with which my feelings surfaced during my training. I did not trust anyone – not my therapist, not the course, not the other students and certainly not myself. I felt certain I would unravel at any moment. Being confronted by the stories of children who, like me, were not prioritised was and continues to be difficult. There have been moments where I have had to work extremely hard to decipher what is my stuff and what is theirs. I have also felt intense feelings of frustration towards parents or carers at times, feeling anger on the child's behalf and perhaps for my own child self too.

I felt significantly tested in personal therapy. There was shame when my therapist asked me questions about my training or asked me about the learning. I thought that she was testing me – to see if I was good enough or knew enough. I feared that she would see me for who I felt I was: a fraud. Despite shame's ability to draw us inwards, shame is inextricably linked to our encounters and experiences with others. Our perception of self is compromised as we compare ourselves, perceiving others as "more than" ourselves. Despite shame's links to our experiences and interactions with others, this is also where we can do the most healing. Reparative processes can take place in our relationship with our therapists.

*I am in the women's refuge today. Seven-year-old Zayn is playing with Thera-putty – pulling and stretching it between his hands. He forms it into a large heavy ball. It is the extra strong tub so it takes a lot of work and effort to manipulate. His mother is over in the corner, we have been doing some therapeutic family play sessions recently. I glance over to see what she is up to. WHACK. The ball hits me square in the nose. My eyes water instantly. I explain I am not for throwing things at. I see him crumble internally. I really want to cry.*

*Zayn spends the rest of the session "controlling" me and his mother with pow-ers. This includes being able to make our "noses" tickle. I wonder if he feels bad about hitting me in the face – he wants it to feel "tickly" rather than hurt. I acknowledge again with him the following week about what happened last ses-sion and remind him about us keeping each other safe and not hurting each other – he squirms uncomfortably. I feel him shutting down and withdrawing. I wonder if I damaged the relationship or ruptured it in some way – was I not gentle or kind enough? Zayn decides he does not want to come to today's session after all.*

I instantly recognised that the incident with Zayn had triggered his own feel-ings of shame and stirred within him a deep-rooted fear – that he is bad, and that he is not wanted. He often makes statements that everyone hates him. I could feel these feelings within me too – a transference? Perhaps. Maybe also my own feelings of inadequacy resurfacing. In the following weeks, I acknowledged how much I enjoyed him coming to play therapy. One day he shared with me that the room made him feel scared because of a spider he had seen in the tent – his deepest phobia. Following that, I armed myself with an empty container to catch the spider whilst he instructed me where to look and helped by shaking the tent roof. At one point, he grasped my hand when he thought he saw one – he had not – and I saw in that moment that the relationship had not ruptured beyond repair after all.

I can relate to Zayn in many ways. I too was an extremely sensitive, imag-inative and playful child. But the older I got the more serious and withdrawn I became. I often felt "silly" at the start of my training. Role-playing felt like a fresh dose of hell each time and the fact that other people seemed to be enjoying it was incredulous. I had forgotten how to be playful, how to let go and be creative. Shame made me hate my child self. I wanted her to disappear. But I had to find a way to reconnect with her, to reassure her and to reaffirm her. Personal therapy is a necessary and painful journey. Thankfully, my therapist gave me many oppor-tunities to be playful. One "homework" I had was to read the "Velveteen Rabbit". This was another part of her helping me to connect with my own inner child and finding a way to empathise with her. Nearing the end of four and a half years in therapy, I had the following dream:

*I dream of a large, ghostly house – full of huge, tall ceilinged, empty rooms. I am trying to say goodbye to someone who is in the house but I can't find them. I wander from room to room, trying to find them. But they are far away. They leave before I can say anything. I get to an attic – and find Scarlett. The little girl from my first placement. She is sat on the floor – surrounded by all of her artwork. We look through the various images together. She turns to me, "I looked for you, but I couldn't find you".*

## Part 5

*The little boy recognised where he was. They were now in the forest by his house. There were many things here – rubbish, old toys and discarded junk. The little boy busied himself with a broken bike – he didn't ask for help fixing it. The spider reflected that the end of a journey could be both sad and exciting. Once the little boy had fixed the bike, he told the spider he knew the way forward.*

## Through and beyond healing

> The good life is a process, not a state of being. It is a direction, not a destination.
>
> (Rogers, 1967: 186)

We often tell parents and carers before starting play therapy to be prepared that things might get worse before they get better. And so it goes for us too. It gets worse because it must. We are not one-dimensional beings, but people with histories and experiences. Play therapy training mirrors the journey taken by our clients, as we move through various stages towards "mastery" (Nordling & Guerney, 1999). We begin as fledglings, exploring and adjusting, integrating new learning and skills. As we work, we are sometimes overcome by an intensity of feelings and memories; rage and regression. Once we have processed and integrated this, we can move towards mastery.

We can learn a lot from our own shame. Understanding it most certainly helps us to recognise it in the clients we work with. Within my own research the common themes associated with shame were identified as a sense of unworthiness, fear of exposure and feelings of disconnection. Orange (1995) highlights that the process of escaping through the isolated world of shame is to connect with others, which in turn risks the possibly of entering into shame once more. Taking risks and speaking out allows us the possibility of discovering something else. As awareness increases, we begin to feel worthy of belonging, we develop a new way of "being". We discover new strategies for dealing with uncomfortable situations and managing relationships. We challenge shame by pushing ourselves forward and not remaining silent.

Had I not studied shame, I would not have been able to distinguish it in those I work with. In the aftermath of her disclosure, I could not recognise that what Scarlett was feeling was shame. I could not see it in myself. I probably would have called it embarrassment. Working with Chloe and Zayn, I can now recognise it and could take steps to try and work through it with them. I see it in the parents and carers I work with who fear they are not good enough; women in the refuge, adoptive parents, grandparents who have their grandchildren via Special Guardianship Orders. Shame hides in many places.

Play therapy training emphasises our need to empathise with people's experiences and see them through a lens of unconditional positive regard. Acceptance and validation from others encourage internal acceptance. When we extend this to ourselves, we can also make peace with ourselves as unperfect beings, viewing ourselves and experiences not just as black and white, but also shades of grey. We do not have to be perfect; we are neither good nor bad, but "good enough" (Winnicott, 1980). Letting go of perfect ideals allows us to truly be ourselves. We have survived our hardships. And our struggles and disappointments can be part of everyday human experience, rather than internalised and blamed on the self.

I believe a multifaceted approach to therapeutic training, which encourages personal therapy and congruence within supervision and other aspects of the course, can provide a space for shame-prone people to begin to develop shame resilience and work towards healing. But if it is not an integral part of students learning, many will never know or understand the depths of shame, nor how to combat it. Through working on my own shame, and discovering ways to manage it, I have much less reluctance to share my vulnerabilities with others and I have found it as a force for others' sharing too.

Shame-prone people struggle with their "sense of self" and working through our shame helps develop a new identity. The training becomes more than just academic and professional growth; it is the catalyst for understanding. The depths of shame and the necessary self-search required to overcome it allow us to connect with the experience. We identify it in others and empathise on a deeper level. We learn that our shame can be a part of our experience without overwhelming it. That it can be a force for connection, understanding and empathy. Our training starts a process of evolution, but there is no endpoint.

Speaking out on my shame meant I had to be brave. And being brave in one area of my life caused it to filter out into others. I was reclusive during my training and it took me a long time to feel connected to my "self" again. In 2020, for my 29th birthday (a day I usually hate and avoid), I completed a 23-mile walk from Box Hill to Seale, Surrey on my own. It took me 7.5 hours. At the end I stood on top of a hill, cried and thought "what a journey!"

## Part 6

*He noticed a beam of sunshine breaking through the clouds above the house. The spider told the little boy that she would be going back to her web. The little boy told the spider that he would miss her greatly. And the spider knew she would miss the little boy too.*

*The little boy and his mother went back into the house. And although the house could still be scary at times and make him feel angry and cross, the shadows did not cause him as much bother anymore. And the little boy found he was able to manage them when they did. He often remembered the spider, and the special journey they had made together, and so he was not so angry or messy or scared anymore.*

All clinical material in this chapter has been anonymised and pseudonymised to protect and maintain the confidentially of those involved.

## References

Adams, M. (2014) *The Myth of the Untroubled Therapist: Private Life, Professional Practice.* London: Routledge. Available at: www.dawsonera.com (Accessed: 19 October 2017).

Alex Linley, P. & Joseph, S. (2007) Therapist Work and Therapists' Positive and Negative Well-Being. *Journal of Social and Clinical Psychology*, 26(3), pp. 385–403. Available at: http://web.ebscohost.com (Accessed: 03 November 2017).

Andrews, B. & Hunter, E. (1997) Shame, Early Abuse, and Course of Depression in a Clinical Sample: A Preliminary Study. *Cognition and Emotion*, 11(4), pp. 373–381. Available at: www.tandfonline.com (Accessed: 13 February 2018).

Badenoch, B. (2008) *Being a Brain-Wise Therapist: A Practical Guide to Interpersonal Neurobiology.* London: W. W. Norton & Company.

Barr, A. (2006) *An Investigation Into the Extent to Which Psychological Wounds Inspire Counsellors and Psychotherapists to Become Wounded Healers, the Significance of These Wounds on Their Career Choice, the Causes of These Wounds and the Overall Significance of Demographic Factors.* MSc Dissertation. University of Strathclyde. Available at: www.thegreenrooms.net (Accessed: 25 October 2017).

Black, R., Curran, D. & Dyer, K. (2013) The Impact of Shame on the Therapeutic Alliance and Intimate Relationships. *Journal of Clinical Psychology*, 69(6), pp. 646–654. Available at: www.ebscohost.com (Accessed: 23 May 2018).

Broucek, F. J. (1991) *Shame and the Self.* New York: The Guilford Press.

Brown, B. (2007) *I Thought It Was Just Me (But It Isn't).* New York: Avery.

Brown, B. (2012) *Daring Greatly: How the Courage to Be Vulnerable Transforms the Way We Live, Love, Parent and Lead.* London: Penguin.

Brown, B., Rondero Hernandez, V. & Villareal, Y. (2011) Connections: A 12-Session Psychoeducational Shame Resilience Curriculum. In: Dearing, R. & Tangney, J. (eds.) *Shame in the Therapy Hour* (pp. 355–371). Washington: American Psychological Association. Available at: www.ebscohost.com (Accessed: 2 March 2018).

Clough, M. (2014) Atoning Shame. *Feminist Theology*, 23(1), pp. 6–17. Available at: http://journals.sagepub.com (Accessed: 15 February 2018).

Dearing, R., Stuewig, J. & Tangney, J. (2005) On the Importance of Distinguishing Shame from Guilt: Relations to Problematic Alcohol and Drug Use. *Addictive Behaviours*, 30(7), pp. 1392–1404. Available at: www.researchgate.net (Accessed: 15 February 2018).

Earley, J. (2000) *Interactive Group Therapy: Integrating Interpersonal, Action-oriented, and Psychodynamic Approaches.* [Google Books] Philadelphia, PA: Brunner/Mazel.

Epstein, N. & Falconier, M. (2011) Shame in Couple Therapy: Helping to Heal the Intimacy Bond. In: Dearing, R. & Tangney, J. (eds.) *Shame in the Therapy Hour* (pp. 167–193). Washington: American Psychological Association. Available at: www.ebscohost.com (Accessed: 2 March 2018).

Gans, J. & Weber, R. (2000) The Detection of Shame in Group Psychotherapy: Uncovering the Hidden Emotion. *International Journal of Group Psychotherapy*, 50(3), pp. 381–396. Available at: www.tandfonline.com (Accessed: 2 June 2018).

Gerhardt, S. (2004) *Why Love Matters: How Affection Shapes a Baby's Brain.* Hove: Brunner-Routledge, Dawson Era. Available at: www.dawsonera.com (Accessed: 6 January 2017).

Gilbert, P. (2011) Shame in Psychotherapy and the Role of Compassion Focused Therapy. In: Dearing, R. & Tangney, J. (eds.) *Shame in the Therapy Hour* (pp. 325–354). Washington: American Psychological Association. Available at: www.ebscohost.com (Accessed: 3 June 2018).

Greenberg, L. & Iwakabe, S. (2011) Emotion-Focused Therapy and Shame. In: Dearing, R. & Tangney, J. (eds.) *Shame in the Therapy Hour* (pp. 69–90). Washington: American Psychological Association. Available at: www.ebscohost.com (Accessed: 2 April 2018).

Hahn, W. (2001) The Experience of Shame in Psychotherapy Supervision. *Psychotherapy: Theory, Research, Practice, Training*, 38(3), pp. 272–282. Available at: http://web.ebscohost.com (Accessed: 23 October 2017).

Hedman, E., Ström, P., Stünkel, A. & Mörtberg, E. (2013) Shame and Guilt in Social Anxiety Disorder: Effects of Cognitive Behavior Therapy and Association with Social Anxiety and Depressive Symptoms. *PLoS One*, 8(4). Available at: http://web.ebscohost.com (Accessed: 11 March 18).

Jung, C. (1963) Psychiatric Activities. In: Jaffé, A. (ed.) *Memories, Dreams, Reflections.* London: Collins and Routledge & Kegan Paul.

Ladany, N., Hill, C., Corbett, M. & Nutt, E. (1996) Nature, Extent, and Importance of What Psychotherapy Trainees Do Not Disclose to Their Supervisors. *Journal of Counseling Psychology*, 43(1), pp. 10–24. Available at: http://web.ebscohost.com (Accessed: 20 October 2017).

Ladany, N., Klinger, R. & Kulp, L. (2011) Therapist Shame: Implications for Therapy and Supervision. In: Dearing, R. L. & Tangney, J. P. (eds.) *Shame in the Therapy Hour* (pp. 307–322). Washington: American Psychological Association. Available at: http://web.ebscohost.com (Accessed: 2 March 2017).

Lewis, H. B. (1971) *Shame and Guilt in Neurosis.* New York: International Universities Press, Inc.

Macaskill, N. & Macaskill, A. (1992) Psychotherapists-in-Training Evaluate Their Personal Therapy: Results of a UK Survey. *British Journal of Psychotherapy*, 9(2), pp. 133–138. Available at: http://web.ebscohost.com (Accessed: 23 October 2017).

McEwan, J. & Duncan, P. (1993) Personal Therapy in the Training of Psychologists. *Canadian Psychology/Psychologie Canadienne*, 34(2), pp. 186–197. Available at: http://web.ebscohost.com (Accessed: 23 October 2017).

McHenry, S. (1994) When the Therapist Needs Therapy: Countertransference Issues and Failures in the Treatment of the Borderline Personality Disorder. *Psychotherapy: Theory, Research, Practice, Training*, 31(4), pp. 557–570. Available at: http://web.ebscohost.com (Accessed: 19 October 2017).

Miller, A. (1990) *Banished Knowledge: Facing Childhood Injuries.* New York: Doubleday. Available at: https://books.google.co.uk (Accessed: 12 April 2018).

Nathanson, D. (1992) *Shame and Pride: Affect, Sex, and the Birth of the Self.* New York: Norton.

Nordling, W. & Guerney, L. (1999) Typical Stages in the Child-Centered Play Therapy Process. *The Journal of the Professional Counsellor*, 14(1), pp. 17–24.

Orange, D. (1995) *Emotional Understanding: Studies in Psychoanalytic Epistemology.* New York: Guilford Press.

Rogers, C. (1967) *A Therapist's View on Psychotherapy: On Becoming a Person.* London: Constable.

Sanftner, J. & Tantillo, M. (2011) Body Image and Eating Disorders: A Compelling Source of Shame for Women. In: Dearing, R. & Tangney, J. (eds.) *Shame in the Therapy Hour* (pp. 277–303). Washington: American Psychological Association. Available at: www.ebscohost.com (Accessed: 2 March 2018).

Schoenleber, M. & Gratz, K. (2018) Self-Acceptance Group Therapy: A Transdiagnostic, Cognitive-Behavioral Treatment for Shame. *Cognitive and Behavioral Practice*, 25(1), pp. 75–86. Available at: www.sciencedirect.com/ (Accessed: 5 June 2018).

Schore, A. N. (1991) Early Superego Development: The Emergence of Shame and Narcissistic Affect Regulation in the Practicing Period. *Psychoanalysis and Contemporary Thought*, 14(2), pp. 187–250. Available at: www.pep-web.com (Accessed: 18 March 2018).

Schore, A. N. (1994) *Affect Regulation and the Origin of the Self: The Neurobiology of Emotional Development*. Hillsdale, NJ: Erlbaum.

Shahar, B., Doron, G. & Szepsenwol, O. (2015) Childhood Maltreatment, Shame-Proneness and Self-Criticism in Social Anxiety Disorder: A Sequential Mediational Model. *Clinical Psychology & Psychotherapy*, 22(6), pp. 570–579. Available at: www.ebscohost.com (Accessed: 16 March 2018).

Shapiro, E. & Powers, T. (2011) Shame and the Paradox of Group Therapy. In: Dearing, R. & Tangney, J. (eds.) *Shame in the Therapy Hour* (pp. 115–135). Washington: American Psychological Association. Available at: www.ebscohost.com (Accessed: 2 March 2018).

Stuewig, J., Tangney, J., Kendall, S., Folk, J., Meyer, C. R. & Dearing, R. (2015) Children's Proneness to Shame and Guilt Predict Risky and Illegal Behaviors in Young Adulthood. *Child Psychiatry and Human Development*, 46(2), pp. 217–227. Available at: http://web.ebscohost.com (Accessed: 13 March 2018).

Tangney, J. & Dearing, R. (2002) *Shame and Guilt*. New York: Guilford Press.

Timm, T. & Blow, A. (1999) Self-of-the-Therapist Work: A Balance Between Removing Restraints and Identifying Resources. *Contemporary Family Therapy: An International Journal*, 21(3), pp. 331–351. Available at: http://web.ebscohost.com (Accessed: 20 October 2017).

Webb, M., Heisler, D., Call, S., Chickering, S. & Colburn, T. (2007) Shame, Guilt, Symptoms of Depression, and Reported History of Psychological Maltreatment. *Child Abuse and Neglect*, 31(11–12), pp. 1143–1153. Available at: www.sciencedirect.com (Accessed: 18 March 2018).

Williams, M. (2004) *The Original Velveteen Rabbit*. London: Egmont.

Winnicott, D. (1980) *Playing and Reality*. Harmondsworth: Penguin.

Wurmser, L. (1981) *The Mask of Shame*. Baltimore: John Hopkins University Press.

# Chapter 6

# Present without presence

## Supporting the dissociative child in play therapy

*Genene Grubb*

*Altogether the trauma is unbearable. To survive, the child must break it apart into pieces, pieces that can never be allowed to reconnect. In this way trauma works like a shattered mirror, reflecting the child's broken life and shattered identity.*

(Gil, in Kagan, 2014: 34)

## Introduction

As play therapists, we are often called upon to work with children who have experienced early and enduring trauma. Because sensory fragments of such traumatic memory can intrude into the present (Van Der Kolk, 2014), they can literally be re-experienced inside the playroom and this enables us to observe and experience the myriad psychological and physiological processes which consequently emerge. One such process may be that of dissociation, which Van Der Kolk (2014: 66) describes as being "the essence of trauma". Working within the settings and systems that we do as play therapists, we find ourselves in a uniquely privileged position; bearing witness to the range of experiences, feelings and processes brought to us in playrooms, family consultations, professionals' meetings and, more recently, online sessions. It seems then that if we are to be equipped with the understanding and skills necessary to support traumatised children, it is vital we possess the ability to recognise the signs of, and capacity to therapeutically work with, the dissociative mechanisms which have enabled these children to survive.

My own awareness of such dissociative processes continues to develop as I meet and work with more children and families in play therapy. However, in addition to an ever-growing belief in its clinical applicability, my curiosity around dissociation began long before I became a play therapist and stems from some of my own lived experiences, which were perhaps the catalyst for pursuing this career path in child therapy. Dissociation as a psychological mechanism has fascinated me for a number of years, and truthfully, perplexed and, in some moments, frightened me too. However, my introduction to some of the more debilitating and

DOI: 10.4324/9781003017271-6

extreme effects of trauma-related dissociation were observed whilst working as a support worker in a psychiatric intensive care unit for adolescents.

I am instantaneously taken aback for the first time I was called to respond to a young person who was experiencing a vivid and terrifying flashback in one of the wards. There were already several support workers present in this child's room, but due to the nature of this incident and the level of distress this young person was experiencing, it necessitated further support. From the moment I stepped onto the ward, I could hear a child screaming and rushed down the corridor to witness this terrified young person crying, punching, kicking, throwing furniture, scratching at her face and arms whilst fiercely attempting to fight off those who approached her. It was my first week on the job and though I felt incapacitated by an awareness of a very real risk to my own safety, with no idea what I should do and how to help, what I most remember is the power of the feeling evoked within me upon hearing her desperate pleas for whatever horror she was re-experiencing, and whoever was causing it, to stop.

I can think back to many instances where I was confronted by a young person who's past and present became confused, catapulted back to those feelings of despair. Trapped in the trauma of their childhood, terrified and helpless or lost in an uncontrollable dissociative fit of rage. In nearly all these situations, where it had escalated to the point of causing physical harm, we had to rely on restraint, holding the child still on the bed or the floor until the worst passed. Sometimes it would be two of us, sometimes up to four people would be immobilising the arms and legs of a young person. I have often since contemplated the level of training support workers receive when entering such settings and how frightening and confusing this can be to face for the first time. However, more often I think about how frightened and powerless this vulnerable young person must have felt.

Reflecting on my time as a support worker unequipped with the tools to therapeutically manage such incidences of dissociation and solely relying on restraint techniques to keep the adolescents physically safe from harm, I have since thought about the repercussions and cost of this response to their distress. It seems likely that there could have been other more effective and therapeutic ways to work with them, which ensured not just their physical safety, but their psychological safety too, rather than decisions based on the reactive thinking of a group of often young, unsure, inexperienced support workers with limited training and understanding around trauma. On most occasions, I did not know what I would be responding to when the alarms went off and there was often no context for the events preceding the incident, so decisions had to be made quickly and without much opportunity to think and plan.

Witnessing the long-lasting effects of traumatic childhood experiences on these adolescents in a clinical setting led me to wonder how such experiences might manifest themselves in the playroom when working with traumatised children in play therapy. My personal responses to such experiences have also caused me to believe that therapists' own feelings and reactions to dissociation may be an integral part of working with it therapeutically. This was substantiated during my play therapy training, when undertaking my placement with families affected by domestic violence, and more specifically, children who have been exposed to significant developmental trauma. For this reason, I decided to embark upon a small-scale qualitative research project designed to capture the subjective experiences of professionals working in the field of play therapy and provide valuable insights into work conducted with dissociation in the playroom, in a way not yet addressed within the existing literature.

The importance of researching this chosen area was not solely highlighted by personal motivations, but crucially, by the lack of literature available on dissociation not only within a play therapy context, but also among other creative therapeutic disciplines. Whilst some documentation of child dissociation exists, research has still lagged behind that of adults (Silberg & Dallam, 2010). A large proportion of the literature available pertains to the clinical assessment of dissociation which, though important, fails to capture the "felt" experiences and reality of working with dissociative children, which perhaps relies less on clinical terminology and criteria. An exploration of some of the thinking and theory around dissociation is outlined in a review of the literature below.

## What is dissociation?

Dissociation appears to exist on a continuum, ranging from regularly experienced states such as daydreaming or complete absorption in a book or film to the kind of dissociative states which cause a disruption in the normal integrative functions of a person's consciousness or even identity (Putnam, 1989). This abnormal dissociation can, however, provide a protective function. James (1989) argues that "defensive dissociation" in children can allow them to function in difficult environments by cutting off overwhelming memories, feelings, thoughts and sensations.

When exposed to extremely threatening situations, be it neglect, intrusion of the body or dangerous surroundings, young infants can rarely flee or effectively fight off such threats. One way that they can keep themselves psychologically "safe" from what is happening and survive overwhelming and potentially repetitive fright is to place space between themselves and the presenting danger (Wieland, 2015). Dissociation is a common survival-focused response to such extreme stressors and appears to be driven by the most primitive brain systems (Perry, 2017). During dissociation, the brain prepares the body for injury, heart rate slows, blood is kept away from extremities and endogenous opioids are released, which kills pain and produces a calm sense of psychological distance from what is occurring (Perry, 2017).

This separation relieves intense stress and anxiety and may be repeated when danger reappears (Wieland, 2015). In time, it can become a regular pattern of responses to frightening or anxiety provoking situations, particularly for those children and adults who have been abused, neglected or terrorised (Silberg, 2013). Without the coping mechanisms to independently self-soothe or protect themselves, nor the mobility to seek another adult for comfort or escape fearful or stressful situations, very young children are more disposed to dissociation (Perry, 2001).

This process involves a compartmentalisation of experience, in which cognitive, emotional or sensory aspects of antecedent events are split from awareness (Dutra et al., 2009). The resulting fragmentation of consciousness can result in thoughts, sensations and images being uprooted from experience and may later impair a person's ability to process and reflect on these states as ones "owned" by themselves (Bromberg, 1998). This lack of integration prevents a comprehensive narrative of the experience developing.

The extreme end of the dissociative continuum is the development of dissociative identity disorder whereby a person completely separates off these disowned thoughts, feelings and sensations into segregated "self-states" with individual states of consciousness or awareness (Waters, 2016). These states may be identified as helpers, protectors, younger regressed self-states or even hostile introjected parts resembling the abuser (Potgieter-Marks, 2012). The child may experience these dissociative states as controlling, helpful, scary or conflicting and might express hearing them fighting or giving messages. (ESTD, 2017).

## How do dissociative defences develop?

As previously stated, there is a continuum on which dissociation functions from the nonpathological to the pathological. Pathological dissociation involves some degree of "structural division" within the self, which causes disturbances in perception, memory, consciousness and perhaps identity (Waters, 2016). There exists a correlation between pathological dissociation and complex trauma (Kisiel et al., 2013), defined as "both children's exposure to multiple traumatic events, usually of an invasive, interpersonal nature, and the wide-ranging, long-term impact of this exposure" (National Child Traumatic Stress Network [NCTSN], 2007: 34). Severity of symptomology has been linked to long-standing trauma, which occurs over multiple critical developmental periods (English et al., 2005).

Van Der Kolk (1987) suggests that the profound effects of such uncontrollable and frightening experiences on younger children, whose cognitive functions and nervous systems are not yet fully developed, means they may be the most vulnerable to damage from childhood trauma. Such early trauma can lead to global impairment and perhaps a reliance on primitive processes, such as dissociation. A child's sense of vulnerability and helplessness will also increase if abuse continues over time, as will the opportunities to utilise and refine these survival mechanisms (Gil, 1991).

There are varying ideas around the development of dissociative symptomology following trauma, but Mann and Sanders (1994) reviewed contemporary models of dissociative aetiology and outlined key common characteristics. Firstly, they all understood dissociation as a normal defence mechanism available in varying degrees in response to overwhelmingly painful, stressful or terrifying scenarios.

Further, the individual differences in the capacity to dissociate are partly biologically or genetically determined, and this capacity is greatest during childhood. It seems that family relationship patterns can also positively influence ability to dissociate or foster overreliance on dissociation. For example, Braun's (1986) 3-P model of developmental factors specifically highlighted how frequent exposure to an unpredictable and inconsistently stressful environment, where the same behaviour may be received in both a loving and abusive way at different times, can predispose children to dissociate.

One theory about why the brain might develop such defences is the affect avoidance theory of dissociation posited by Silberg (2013), who suggested that because affects associated with frightening stimuli are aversive, children block them out to relieve their vulnerability. Over time, these patterns of avoidance, which may generalise to other non-traumatising situations which similarly trigger the original negative affect, activate conditioned, automatic avoidance responses, which become increasingly outside of awareness (Silberg, 2017).

Braun (1988) also expanded on this theoretical model of the aetiology of dissociation by integrating the cognitive model of state-dependent learning. According to this model, a child who is in a state of increased neuropsychophysiological (NPP) arousal and dissociates during a traumatic incident may only retrieve the memories of this experience when in a similar state of NPP arousal. Over repeated episodes of dissociation, or compartmentalising, during NPP states, Braun (1988) argued that dissociated material, such as associated knowledge, memories and affective, behavioural, physiological and sensory responses become linked together.

Other autonomic and unconscious processes that may explain the presence of dissociation come from extensive research conducted by Porges (2011). Porges discovered a third branch of the Autonomic Nervous System (ANS), the social engagement nervous system, where previously it was believed there was only the sympathetic and the parasympathetic. This third division is the most advanced branch and promotes maternal bonding and connection with others by fostering social communication through facial expressions, vocalisation and listening.

According to Porges (2011), these systems function hierarchically. In response to threat and failure to be rescued, the highest branch of the ANS, the social engagement system, shuts down, automatically activating the division below, the sympathetic nervous system. This system is responsible for enabling mobility to scavenge food and defend against threats and also triggers the fight-or-flight responses, increasing heart rate and pumping blood to the muscles. When an individual is able to neither defend themselves nor flee, the sympathetic nervous system shuts down and the parasympathetic nervous system becomes active. This branch operates at the most primitive level, associated with primal survival strategies, and initiates a freeze response (Waters, 2016). In this last attempt at survival, a general shutdown of the body occurs, resulting in feigning death, immobilisation and/or dissociation (Porges, 2011). This automatic, hierarchical functioning of the ANS can help make sense of a child's response to abuse. Initially, their social engagement system is violated by the abuser and can no longer operate. The child, unable to seek support or feasibly fight or flee, unconsciously engages the most primitive and primal automatic survival strategies, freezing and dissociating.

Alternative research suggests that attachment style and the quality of family relationships, specifically the mother-infant dyad, is a predictor or dissociative symptomology. Avoidant and disorganised attachments may predispose children to have dissociative responses to trauma (Barach, 1991; Liotti, 1999a, 1999b) and longitudinal studies have even demonstrated that these attachment styles can predict later dissociation in teenagers (Ogawa et al., 1997). Freyd (1996) further expanded on this to emphasise the significance of betrayal within the attachment relationship as an indicator of reliance on survival mechanisms, such as dissociation. He proposes that betrayal by a trusted caregiver initiates a particularly complex process because the child relies on their caregivers for survival and cannot, therefore, instigate the normal response to betrayal, which would involve experiencing pain and avoiding contact with the betrayer. If abused children withdrew from their primary caregiver, their life would be put in even greater danger; therefore, Freyd (1996) suggests that survival is prioritised and consequently, victims of betrayal trauma learn to deal with this unavoidable conflict through internal disconnection, such as dissociation, instead of external avoidance. However, a child abused outside of the family home may be more able to turn to their family for protection and support and project the "badness" outside their survival system (Gil, 1991).

Importantly, this literature doesn't account for the healthy use of dissociation in our day-to-day lives. As previously mentioned, it offers a positive function in helping to detach and distance oneself in a way that can allow for helpful processing of feelings and experiences (Putnam, 1989). One way this is extremely useful is for the child in the playroom, who uses narratives and characters to explore their own self-concept and feelings at a safe distance, through the symbolic world of pretend. Though these valuable dissociative processes are available to us all, the literature predominantly focuses on the pathological side of dissociation and may miss some key insights into the beneficial work conducted in therapy.

## Recognising dissociation in the playroom

Adler-Tapia and Settle (2008) suggest that therapists working with traumatised children should be encouraged to recognise that they will also be working with some degree of dissociation. They emphasise the importance of understanding dissociative symptomology because, although children who have experienced distressing or traumatic events often present with dissociative qualities, it is crucial not to pathologise children's natural imagination and propensity to engage in fantasy but instead to consider the continuum of normal development in children. For example, The Child and Adolescent Committee of the European Society on Trauma and Dissociation (ESTD) (2017) indicate that dissociative children may readily transition into fantasy or prefer to alternate between different fantasy characters when completing tasks to the extent that it has a negative influence on their general performance. This differs from "normative" use of fantasy whereby the child enjoys engaging in fantasy play and can quickly move back to reality and assume appropriate responsibility.

Assessment can help ascertain how much a child relies on dissociation as a coping mechanism, especially after the traumatic experiences necessitating it have ceased, and whether it is problematic, causing difficulties in the child's life and changing the course of normal development. Waters (2016) emphasises that familiarity with the warning signs of dissociation in children is fundamental if they are to receive appropriate treatment and care and to prevent misdiagnosis. Dissociative children are particularly vulnerable to repeated intervention failures and may experience helplessness, shame and worthlessness for their lack of progress. Waters (2016) suggests that therapists should be mindful if there is a history or childhood trauma and assess the level of caregiver support received. If low, then to ascertain what the child did themselves to manage in response to frightening experiences. Children who have found survival and attachment at odds, due to experiencing abuse in primary attachment relationships, often use dissociation to cope with and survive the resulting distress.

Waters (2016) characterised some indicators of dissociation which may specifically be observed in therapy. Glazed looks, eyes rolling back/fluttering, daydreaming or blanking out may be common. Clients can become startled when the therapist speaks or moves, or display extreme changes in mood, noticeable behavioural changes in expression, posture, voice, handwriting or dress. Dramatic changes in preference for activities, contradictory statements in short succession, unexplained confusion or discrepancies in stories or refuting witnessed behaviour, resulting in children being accused of lying, were also highlighted. According to Perry (2006), dissociation may manifest as a blank, noncommunicative response, foetal rocking, yawning or even falling asleep in response to overwhelming distress. Children may also act out the dissociation by taking on the persona of an animal. Adler-Tapia and Settle illustrate a case in which a child client undergoing Eye Movement Desensitisation and Reprocessing (EMDR) became a startled, hypervigilant deer moving around the room on all fours (2008: 267).

## Working with dissociation in play therapy

Increasing literature is being published within the field outlining treatment interventions for dissociative children (Gomez, 2013; Silberg, 2013). Specific methods may differ across disciplines, but some key aspects are common to all. Fundamentally, the literature suggests that physical and psychological safety is paramount in the therapeutic environment, enabling children to re-establish feelings of trust, reconnection and security (Myrick & Green, 2014). Consistent and predictable environments allow children to relax their defences and trust that their needs will be met (Waters, 2016) and, in line with child-centred theory (Landreth, 2012; Rogers, 1951), unconditional positive regard and implementing necessary limit setting can powerfully facilitate the development of a sense of safety. With a fear of being judged or rejected, traumatised children are especially sensitive to adult responses and Waters (2016) suggests that an open, inquisitive, empathic and collaborative approach is vital. When children feel therapists are genuinely interested without judgement, their fears and dissociative defences will diminish (Waters, 2016).

In fact, it is suggested through Herman's (1992) three-stage treatment model for dissociative adults that the first stage, stabilisation, is imperative if the client is to begin any successful trauma processing as they must be able to cope with the stress linked to these traumatic memories and have capacity to think and evaluate. Wieland (2015) outlines this phase specifically in the treatment of children as creating safety, stability in daily life, psycho-education and handling triggers. Importantly, Herman's model recommends that interventions in the stabilisation stage should be informed by the neuro-sequential model of therapeutics (NMT) (Perry, 2006), mirroring the development of the brain. This framework highlights the powerful association created in utero between maternal heart rate and the need for patterned, repetitive, rhythmic sensory input to soothe and regulate the brain and reach the poorly organised neural networks involved in the stress response (Perry, 2011). These rhythmic, self-nurturing experiences allow a child to be fully present in the moment, connecting to their senses, bodily sensations, movement and any emotions provoked (Wieland, 2015).

In instances where children not only become numb to the process but also lose a connection with the therapist and therapy room, Adler-Tapia and Settle (2008) advise that the child can no longer engage in therapy because dissociation likely inhibits processing altogether and risks re-traumatisation. Treatment should, therefore, be stopped, and the clinician should support the child to reconnect to the therapist and the room using grounding techniques. For example, the therapist may stomp their feet, move their body or gently toss a pillow to the child to encourage them to reconnect with their body and the safety of the room. Crucially, when working with children who dissociate, they recommend spending significant time with the child and parents in the preparation phase, prior to treatment, providing psychoeducation on dissociation and emotional literacy and building skills and techniques around affect regulation, mindfulness and body awareness in order to keep the child's body engaged and stay connected during therapy. Adler-Tapia and Settle also recommend creating with the child safe/calm places in the office or providing a transitional object, such as notebook or blanket, to use when they are distressed and to also create a "sense of object permanency with the therapist" (2008: 270).

Liana Lowenstein (2014), a registered social worker and certified play therapist, also offers some practical advice for addressing child dissociation in sessions, drawing on other available literature (Blaustine & Kinniburgh, 2010; Linehan, 1993; The International Society for the Study of Dissociation, 2003). In response to instances of dissociation, she suggests speaking calmly and reassuring the child that nothing bad is happening and they are safe, empathising with them, "you look scared, I'm sorry the siren scared you" (Lowenstein, 2014: 1) and encourage grounding techniques, such as "I spy", naming things they can see, tapping their feet ten times or naming the days of the week. Once children become re-embodied, Lowenstein recommends physical activity, such as star jumps, dancing, drumming, running on the spot or yoga. In more recent literature, The Child and Adolescent Committee of the European Society on Trauma and Dissociation (ESTD) (2017) suggests incorporating safe smells, chewy/crunchy food, sucking lollies or bottles and introducing breathing exercises. For regressive dissociative states, having safe and nurturing touch through massage, if tolerated, being rocked in a hammock, being fed or singing self-made songs can soothe and support the child.

Also promoted within the treatment literature are approaches directly targeting dissociative symptomology. Gil (1991), another prominent contributor to the play therapy literature, proposed a step-by-step technique for addressing dissociation in children. She highlighted the need to carefully develop a developmentally appropriate, normalising language around dissociation for the child and ask them to give their unique process a name. Assessing patterns and triggers for dissociation is also important for the child to recognise what is happening to them and why. Gil (1991) noted that some precipitants to dissociative responses are physical pain, anger, sexual arousal, shame and longing. Whilst explaining how dissociation is adaptive, she encourages therapists to provide healthy alternative ways of coping to enable the child to feel in control. These coping strategies prevent the identified emotions being avoided or repressed, for example, by externalising them through drawing and open conversation until the child is more able to tolerate discussion and intolerable emotions are desensitised.

Offering some alternative views, though not a comprehensive treatment plan, Triplett (2007) advocates therapists not to interfere with the dissociative child unless they or the child are at risk. She argues that the needs and emotions expressed should be given the same time, care and attention as non-dissociative material, though playroom limits still apply. Triplett suggests that dissociative behaviour can provide valuable insight into the inner world of the client and asserts that children dissociate for a reason and counsellors should respond to the need behind the dissociation. Though, similarly to Gil, Triplett proposes that it can be addressed using normalising language afterwards.

Wieland (2015) suggests that the playroom itself also serves to mitigate dissociative tendencies in posttraumatic children as the child's body is often soothed by play materials and activities, which ground the child to the here and now. Furthermore, Triplett (2007) proposes that determining children's repertoire for self-soothing and bringing elements of this into the playroom, such as a special teddy or blanket, and asking them to create a "safe space" can convey therapists' confidence in the child's ability to create their own safety.

Similarly to Gil, Triplett highlights the importance of contextual factors in gaining a comprehensive understanding, such as frequency, timing and intensity of play and dissociative behaviours. She emphasises working closely with caregivers to help them understand the function of dissociation and create special rituals, which communicate safety, caring, appropriate touch and non-demanding love to strengthen attachment relationships. Equally, Triplett agrees the ultimate goal is to build other coping resources to empower the child with agency and choice over how to manage the situation.

Although the literature available on the indicators of dissociation is very helpful, it is important to remember the uniqueness of each individual's response to trauma and the intricate nuances of behaviour that can be so easily missed by practitioners. To think a child will present with distinct, predictable and recognisable patterns is over-simplistic and it may be that clinical experience has the most significant influence on accurate and appropriate diagnosis and response. Perhaps, building on the commentary available of therapists' personal experiences will shed light on working with dissociative children in play therapy and help less experienced therapists know what to look for in children who dissociate and which questions to ask to ensure nothing important is missed.

## Personal impact of research and implications

Upon conducting my research project, I realised that what appears to be distinctly missing from the literature is an account from the view of the perceiving, receiving, responding and attuning other; the therapist who bears witness and, at times, joins the child in synchrony, two minds linking up unconsciously. Or, perhaps, the account of the therapist who is triggered by the child's traumatic play and enters their own altered or detached state within the therapy room. It is experiential reporting, such as this, which I hoped to expand on by capturing the phenomenon of child dissociation from the perspective of those who have lived experience of it and hopefully, indirectly, capture the experience of the child in the room. However, what emerged from listening to the stories of experienced therapists went far beyond academic pursuit. It proved to be a fascinating, illuminating and comforting endeavour through which I was able to find many commonalities amongst the experiential process of the therapists, learn from their experience and gain a more personal, accessible account of dissociation in the playroom and its effects. The opportunity to reflect upon my own process of taking on the challenge of a project such as this proved also to be hugely valuable.

Revisiting the literature in the process of writing this chapter has served as a strong reminder of the pain, suffering and helplessness intrinsic to the development of the most chronic forms of dissociation. It was a difficult material to be analysing in such detail and I recall having many powerful emotional responses to the profound and enduring childhood trauma captured within the moving depictions of the work conducted by experienced play therapists within the field. Being aware of the strength of such reactions elicited simply by reading these words on a page only impresses on me the emotional toll we as therapists take on when working with this level of hurt and vulnerability. For me, there were also some parallels to be drawn with the dissociative child, in my response to the colossal task of completing this research project. Many times, I found myself frozen in a state of helplessness, unable to open my laptop and bring words to the page.

Importantly, the learning I have taken with me, both practical and personal, can be understood within the context of the five key themes illuminated within my research. These insights have, and continue to have, resonance within my own practice to this day. The first of which seems potentially self-evident but is important to address as it had a clear effect on the therapeutic response to dissociation and has since influenced my own. This is the therapists' own understanding of dissociation. There appeared to be some variability in the definition and use of dissociation provided by participants, which may be influenced by several factors, such as years of experience and trauma-heavy caseloads. Some participants, for example, described themselves as adopting a wider definition of dissociative processes, which was not solely linked to pathology, later on in their practice. This also determined the frequency at which therapists described themselves to have witnessed dissociation in the playroom.

I believe I came to the project myself with a very narrow view of dissociation, typical of a pathological description you may find in the diagnostic criteria of a mental health disorder. What came out of each conversation with these therapists was a greater understanding and respect for the processes, which have helped these children survive and navigate the incredibly challenging circumstances in which they found themselves; a means by which they were able to protect the psyche from "falling apart" and prevent further psychological trauma. Importantly, I felt less fearful of it, knowing that, perhaps in its widest sense, we see it each and every day in our therapy rooms. If dissociation can offer a child the opportunity to detach from, or split off, intolerable aspects of the self and bring them to the fore through characters in play in order not to ignore or lose these parts altogether, then perhaps this process of disconnection and detachment can eventually facilitate healthier integration of the self, even for children with severe detachment.

Therapeutically, this ongoing journey may be about working with children to help them stay within the safe and healthy spectrum of dissociation. Within this psychic space, they might use detachment positively, experiencing mindlessness, separating their own experience in a way that is digestible and safe through the disguise of storytelling. Or, utilising sensory materials to induce a meditative disconnect from reality, which may serve to soothe and regulate, but could still trigger in the therapist a strong sense that the child is no longer available or present in the room in the same way.

In these instances, it may be important not to "jump in" too early. There are times I have been primed and ready to intervene when a child pauses, becomes quiet or looks like they are shutting down, but in actuality they may be working really hard within themselves to consolidate something that's just been realised. In this way, it is something to be worked with and not against, being open to the possibility that a child is entering a more reflective state through retreating further into themselves and simply holding this space for them.

It does, however, appear crucial that therapists have awareness of the point at which dissociation becomes a pathological issue. The decision to intervene then depends on the level of distress it appears to cause to the child or the extent to which the therapist feels they need to be reached. For example, dissociation by fantasy could be exactly where the child needs to be in that moment, but it can also become problematic, becoming so rigid, the child no longer seems to be experiencing any joy from those fantasies and qualitatively differing from typical imaginative play, which may otherwise be animated, purposeful and non-distressing. However, such abstract intuitions are difficult to define in concrete terms and offer dependable guidance around. It seems then that we must rely heavily on our clinical judgement to ascertain how we might be aware of, and respond to, dissociation. The weight of this responsibility was a particular source of anxiety for me, and I am grateful to have gained further self-compassion through this project, knowing that this anxiety around the management of "unhealthy" dissociation was also felt by other, more experienced therapists.

Ascertaining triggers and precursors of dissociative activity through the research has been particularly helpful when thinking about how to plan for and conduct sessions. The findings from my research highlighted important thinking around preparing toys, the therapeutic space and the way in which therapists interact with traumatised children. Helpfully, common triggers were identified within my research under the following categories: environmental triggers, such as the space itself, the time boundary and outside intrusions; relational triggers, which occur when something within the therapist and child interaction may elicit a dissociative response; internal triggers, such as bodily sensations, physiological states or alterations in body temperature, which might be associated with the child's internal state at the time of experiencing the initial stress; and physical/activity-based triggers, such as certain toys, role-plays or the process of creating something.

This leaves a lot of scope due to the uniqueness of each child's experiences, memories and "invisible" physiological triggers, which may be present within them. These findings highlighted a lack of predictability when working with the "unknown" of child dissociation, leading to a considerable increase in the anxiety levels of the therapist who must rely largely on their own experience, intuition and knowledge of, and relationship with, the child to therapeutically manage this in the room. I hold these important considerations in mind when I am setting up a therapy session and evaluating a therapy kit for the child. It seems there is no concrete way to determine if a toy will trigger a child and perhaps it is less about removing certain toys for all children but understanding the individual history and experiences of each child and feeling prepared should dissociation be triggered within a session. Toys and activities to help a child regulate are particularly important here, but I have also gained awareness of the potency contained within any toy, material or interaction I have with a child.

The findings of my research suggested that therapists can look out for variety of indicators which may inform them about the child's state of integration and dissociation. In addition to the physical presentations outlined in the literature above, rocking, thumb-sucking, rigidity, pausing for extended periods or mindless violence/rage were highlighted. I was interested to hear that verbal signals can include nonsense chatter, babbling, made up words or languages, total silence or the use of confusing identity statements, referring to themselves in third person or not as "I" or "me". Children may also experience memory lapses, appear emotionally detached and apathetic or demonstrate "incomprehensible" narratives or "dreamlike" storytelling within their play.

However, an additional and valuable feature of the work was recognising how the therapist's own internal response to being with the child can act as an incredibly useful gauge of the child's internal state of mind and onset of dissociation. Some internal indicators were described as feeling disconnected from one's own body parts, such as "jelly legs", and not feeling your "whole self", or being unaware of bodily needs, such as needing the toilet or hunger. Therapists may also experience sleepiness, exhaustion, disconnection, a lack of grounding or a "fuzzy brain" resulting from a difficulty processing information or entering a dreamlike, meditative state. This may be a consequence of sharing a space with a completely disconnected child and holding the splitting and detachment, which has occurred within them. Checking in with my own physical self and internal senses is now something I continue to prioritise and reflect on, regardless of whether a child has the potential to dissociate in the room.

Deliberation between therapists about when to step in appears to rest on clinical judgement. If there is a clear sense the child is dissociating in a significant or harmful way, perhaps for some time, then I believe we should be making an effort to try and reach them. However, for some children it seems dissociating can help them to reformulate themselves and manage their difficult feelings. For example, some children described it as tantalising, demonstrating a desire to "go there" because it offers them an escape, or helps them to relax, which can be quite addictive. The consensus was that if a child remains "there" for too long, it can be counterproductive. Therefore, understanding how dissociation may be experienced by the children we work with can help us to respond in the most therapeutically considered way and perhaps provide us with the ability to contextualise otherwise incomprehensible behaviours. Similarly, awareness of the possibility that children may feel shame or embarrassment around dissociation or may be accused of lying for missing instructions or doing things they do not consciously remember can help us demonstrate genuine understanding and normalise these potentially frightening and confusing experiences for the children and their families.

This makes me reflect upon the fundamental feature of the spaces we create, design and psychologically hold, as therapists, to facilitate safety. Of course, this safety is implicit in the practice of therapy, through unconditional positive regard, respecting confidentiality and implementing necessary, predictable limits. However, once a therapist has determined that a child may need help to get out of a detached dissociative state, there are more directive approaches one can take to support the child to feel safe enough to manage. The findings indicated that a combination of audio and physical signals paired with soothing and explicit reassurance of safety is key. The importance of a gentle approach cannot be over-emphasised, whilst both physically and emotionally "staying with the child". Key strategies I have taken forward when working with dissociation involve utilising both physically and mentally engaging processes which ground the child back into their own body as well as their present reality. These include predictable, sequenced games, movement which crosses the midline of the brain and naming physical items in the room. The use of sensory games and toys, such as squeezy objects, music and weighted bean bags, which help to calm the "primal brain" and activate a more associated state whereby the child may be able to think and rationalise once again, is also recommended.

Something that came out of the research project which personally resonated with me, and which others in the field may strongly identify with, was the range of challenges we face when working with such complex psychological processes; challenges which frequently penetrate the safety of the space for both the thera-pist and the child. For example, I often contend with environmental challenges, including noise intrusions or interruptions, when working in "unboundaried" set-tings such as schools. Similarly, balancing time constraints with the fear of a child dissociating at the end of a session without adequate grounding time before they must leave is particularly anxiety inducing as a therapist. Such limitations also impact my ability to effectively write up notes and process what has taken place. Importantly, the unpredictable and unclear nature of dissociation, which can be very subtle and difficult to identify, means that even an exhaustive list of pres-entations would unlikely prepare a therapist for every possible incident of disso-ciation, which could occur in the playroom. This uncertainty may lead to a child picking up on any negative response we communicate non-verbally, interpreting us as being disapproving or rejecting, which can feel quite out of our control. Frustratingly, access to limited information has also played a significant role in impeding my ability to effectively plan for and safeguard children in sessions as well as myself. This suggests that comprehensive assessment is key when work-ing with dissociative children.

Perhaps most challenging are the personal obstacles faced in response to this work, such as unexpected or upsetting feelings, which may interfere with my abil-ity to remain present and available to the child. As practitioners, our own history and unresolved experiences may result in children's play becoming triggering. This is an important awareness to gain as it could severely impact my ability to safely manage the child in session were the content of their play to trigger a sense of detachment. I feel heavily the responsibility and fear, or reality, of not being able to reach a child when in a dissociative state or being unsure how to respond to parallel processes, such as dissociation and hallucination simultaneously. Both situations can quickly induce a sense of paranoia and helplessness. As a newly qualified therapist I know I am particularly susceptible to being over-focused on my own feelings of anxiety, panic and guilt in the face of such challenges, rather than staying with what the child is bringing. Crucially, the possibility of secondary traumatisation when working with these types of complex cases is high and should not be underestimated.

For this reason, the single most important outcome of this research project was highlighting the impact of dissociation on the personal process of the therapist and the importance of self-care. Extreme episodes of dissociation, which I interpret as instances which endure, pose significant risk of harm, or when the child feels "unreachable", were coupled with the most negative emotional descriptors: "awful", "scary", "alarming", "tragic", "deeply sad". Self-doubt seemed highest in relation to these incidents, particularly when experiencing difficulty reaching children during dissociative episodes, resulting in therapists feeling de-skilled, ineffective, useless, powerless, worried and heavily responsible. Dissociation in children can also feel tedious, boring or frustrating to be around or may powerfully project feelings of "vileness", "yuckiness", "violation" or physical nausea within the therapist.

This is important to reflect upon and properly process as it may provoke feelings of dislike towards the child, making it hard to remain open-minded when there is a difficulty separating our own fantasies from those of the dissociative child. These tough experiences are compounded by isolation in the workplace, which can be common within play therapy. When in settings such as this, whether it is a separate building or a classroom in the far corner of a school, I believe it is an important consideration for practicing play therapists to implement contingency plans and know who to contact when necessary. Comprehensive knowledge of the child's history and triggers may also improve our ability to adequately plan for and feel confident in our ability to manage dissociation and reduce anxiety in the playroom.

Critically, managing dissociation involves appropriate guidance and adequate processing and reflection time, supported through good supervision. Personal therapy is also crucial in providing a space for reflecting on and gaining awareness of one's own triggers and exploring the challenges within the work. Specifically, it has supported me in allowing all associated feelings, accepting my personal limits and fostering self-compassion. As well as clinical and social support, I believe the ability to healthily dissociate from work and restore one's inner resources is key to safely navigating the complexities of dissociation in therapeutic work. This demonstrates the importance of making time for self-care activities such as walking, getting out in nature, meeting up with friends, playing music, cooking or watching films. My findings also have implications for therapists working with trauma heavy caseloads and suggest that a balance of varying levels of complexity is vital.

## Dissociation within personal and play therapy experience

When I reflect on my own experiences of dissociation, I am now much more aware of its adaptive purposes rather than it solely being indicative of severe trauma, and perhaps something to be supported out of. During the process of undertaking my research project, I incidentally happened to gain a new, unfortunate perspective on the very phenomenon I was avidly reading about and reporting on. This occurred one evening on my way home from a day of lectures at university when I was standing at the train station waiting for my connection, as I had done hundreds of times. Unusually, this evening I did neither have my headphones in, nor was I engrossed in something on my phone or reading. I was simply looking ahead, lost in thought. Within seconds, a man who stood directly opposite to me on the facing platform suddenly transitioned from his inconspicuous standing position to running at full speed and jumping into the air, where he collided with an oncoming train. There was no one else on my platform and only a couple of people stood far at the other end of his; no one appeared to see what I had just witnessed. What followed was immediate and visceral as though my body had been taken over by someone else. My physical response was to run up and down the platform in the vain attempt to notify a member of staff whilst waving to those on the platform opposite. Some unknown time later, I found myself kneeling on the platform to reassure this man, who had at this point regained consciousness and was screaming in pain, terrified and confused, that help was on its way. Fortunately, it was, and I was soon ushered to the other end of the platform and asked to leave the station.

I am now able to tell this story in one coherent narrative. However, immediately after the incident, I was left with a sense of detachment and the repetitive intrusion of independent sensory fragments, such as a sound and distinct images with nothing in between, akin to a flipbook with many pages missing. Nonetheless, crucially, I had the extra fortune of being able to seek almost immediate support and reassurance from my place of work, which happened to be a crisis intervention service a short walk from the station. Here, I was met by people I knew and trusted. Though I was not yet at the point of making sense of and processing the events of the preceding half hour, I was made to feel cared for and listened to, with a cup of tea in hand. I was also lucky enough to be picked up and taken home by my incredibly supportive father, helping me to feel safe and secure.

One day later, I was able to process some of what occurred in a dissertation supervision session with my supervisor. The day after this, I attended personal therapy where I was provided with an interesting opportunity to reflect upon the event. Initially, I was confused when my therapist asked me from which perspective I viewed the incident in my mind. However, I quickly came to realise that I pictured everything as though spectating from above; none of the images I had available to me were from the perspective of the person doing the running and shouting for help. I was then aided in bringing the experience back into my body to regain some control over it. Throughout this process, I was held, contained and supported in a way most others experiencing this would not be. I am then reminded of the child who has none of these opportunities to integrate and make sense of their experiences at their disposal – helpless and lost without a seeing, hearing, validating other to contain their overwhelming feelings. I can understand how these children must necessarily inhabit a dissociative and depersonalised state of detachment in response to trauma within their day-to-day existence, just to feel able to survive.

My experience of dissociation in therapeutic practice however was not at first obvious in its appearance within the playroom. For one particular child, Jackie (pseudonymised), it was through the gradual unpicking of behaviours and reflecting upon the felt responses manifest in me during these episodes that I, with the experienced eye and ear of my supervisor, was able to understand this child's dissociative processes during her small world play. I believe these signs were initially missed, in part, due to my own feelings of shame and incompetence in my responses to her play. Often, I found myself missing small sections of the session, failing to follow the narrative of her play or being unaware of the time passing. Other times it felt like time was going very slowly and boredom crept in alongside the need to stifle yawns. Yet, no matter how I tracked or attempted to actively engage in her play, Jackie failed to hear me or acknowledge my interjections and appeared to be quite unaware of her surroundings. Perhaps I simply was not concentrating hard enough. My inability to track and keep up with her play often resulted in strong feelings of inadequacy as a therapist and feeling mis-timed and mis-attuned to Jackie.

It seemed I had found myself oscillating between apparent synchronous states of dissociative detachment, to being stuck in repetitive thought patterns and internal confusion triggered by my bewilderment around some of the disorientating, disjointed, incomprehensible narratives that Jackie would often play out within the earlier stages of therapy. At either end, I was unable to be fully present and available to her. After sessions, I was often left feeling that I was not capable of reaching or connecting with her, although I did not know which part of her I was trying to connect with because I was not sure which part of her was available in that moment for connection.

Consequently, I found writing session notes for this child particularly difficult, regularly straining to remember the sequence of play, narratives and characters and duration of each story or questioning whether I had fabricated elements just to make sense of what was unfolding before me. I was just not able to get a solid grip on what was happening for her. Quickly, this became linked to a fear of not being a good enough therapist, impacting my ability to aptly process these experiences in sessions and triggering a need to hide my incompetence around this for some time. How could a good therapist simply forget such powerful portrayals of death and humiliation, deceit and betrayal?

Often stories would centre on the unreliability of relationships and confusion over whether characters were "good" or "bad", victim or perpetrator, saviour or subduer. It was through discussions with my supervisor that we were able to notice that this child entered a dissociative state when engaging in this type of fantasy play as she worked through dilemmas and questions around who and what could be trusted. This may be understood through the context of her early environment and experiences of adults in her life being unpredictable, unsafe to the point of threatening both her life and the life of her mother, disruptive and often unable to follow through on their promises.

After some concerning early sessions where Jackie needed some help to remain regulated and back within the safe spectrum of detachment, the quality of her play began to feel slightly different. It was decided that to over-track or insert myself would have disrupted her thinking and processing. As Jackie's play did not appear to demonstrate the qualities of post-traumatic play as it was not repetitive, seemingly harmful and never become distressing enough to warrant my intervening, we deemed this to be a helpful state of consciousness in which much of her inner processing was done. I soon learned to be okay with not needing to be heard by Jackie, but simply showing my continued presence and acceptance while she played out these important scenes. Over time, her stories became less convoluted, and she began to ask me to participate in the narratives and take on characters until the stories took up less time in sessions, and she began to engage in more creative and focused play, which grounded her to the here and now. Similarly, I felt myself metaphorically re-entering the room during these times, without slipping out of awareness.

If I had continued to try and be the "good therapist" in my mind and track her sufficiently or rescue her from the confusing world she had created, I would not have communicated my patience and respect for her need to play in her own way and I may not have observed the progress I did in her therapy. It has also reinforced the principles underpinning child-centred play therapy of children's inner directional drives and ability to solve their own problems (Axline, 1989). Nevertheless, it proved a huge challenge to sit with this uncertainty for weeks on end, feeling unnoticed and far removed from the play itself, yet trying to continue to have faith in myself and the process.

Since my training, I have frequently reflected upon my ever-present inner critic and how it affected my ability to aptly pick up on the signs available to me. Often it can cause us to, figuratively, close our eyes to important experiences within the therapeutic relationship and perhaps miss moments of real meaning and significance. Instinctively, I took the egocentric view that these apparent "slip-ups" were self-motivated, neglectful or even just born of my own incompetence rather than a window into the child's inner workings and processes. It seems I was quick as a therapist to take away from the rich material and insights the child was providing, attempting to make sense of it by turning it into something more concrete, tangible and comfortable. In other words, finding meaning through a familiar self-filtered, critical lens. Only through supervision was I truly able to separate myself from what really mattered, which was the experience of the child.

## Conclusion

What I found hugely informative about my research project was gaining a sense of how I might contextualise the coping mechanisms available to a child I am assessing and working with, to help indicate whether there is a higher likelihood of dissociation. Common histories emerging from the research have since been reflected in my own work with dissociative cases, particularly those linked to extreme violence within the family system where children are required to take on a protective role. Alternatively, children within emotionally and physically neglectful caregiving environments in which they have had to use projective identification too often deny themselves their authentic feelings and desires because they have to constantly ensure that this system, which they depend on, is not shutting down. To do so, they must appease their caregivers, doing anything to keep them engaged in their lives in order not to die themselves. It seems these children necessarily tend towards using dissociation in a more destructive, pathological way. This can help inform our awareness of where a child is presenting on the dissociative spectrum and may influence our clinical judgement on when to respond or intervene.

However, it appears that the real legacy of this work was identifying signifiers of dissociation within a therapeutic context and highlighting the depth at which therapists are impacted by the children we work with. Dissociation involves a particularly complex and fragile balance between the child and the therapist, requiring skilled attunement to, and awareness of internal states, vulnerabilities and unconscious processes. The implications of this are the fundamental need for self-care and ensuring adequate time and support for processing and reflecting on this work. I believe it is important to emphasise the profound and long-lasting effects that bearing witness to a child responding to or re-experiencing such trauma can have. I am reminded of the intensity of the helplessness and fear I felt that day in the psychiatric ward and how those projected states and feelings can so quickly and sharply be brought to my awareness, both physiologically and emotionally, to this day.

## References

Adler-Tapia, R. & Settle, C. (2008) *EMDR and the Art of Psychotherapy With Children*. New York: Springer Publishing Company.

Axline, V. M. (1989) *Play Therapy*. London: Churchill Livingstone.

Barach, P. M. (1991) Multiple Personality Disorder as an Attachment Disorder. *Dissociation*, 4, pp. 117–123.

Blaustine, M. E. & Kinniburgh, K. M. (2010) *Treating Traumatic Stress in Children and Adolescents: How to Foster Resilience Through Attachment, Self-Regulation, and Competency*. New York: Guildford Press.

Braun, B. G. (1986) Issues in the Psychotherapy of Multiple Personality Disorder. In: Braun, B. G. (ed.) *Treatment of Multiple Personality Disorder* (pp. 1–28). Washington: American Psychiatric Press.

Braun, G. G. (1988) The BASK Model of Dissociation. *Dissociation*, 1(1), pp. 4–23.

Bromberg, P. M. (1998) *Standing in the Spaces. Essays on Clinical Process, Trauma and Dissociation*. Hillsdale: Analytic Press.

Dutra, L., et al. (2009) The Relational Context of Dissociative Phenomena. In: Dell, P. F. & O'Neil, J. A. (eds.) *Dissociation and the Dissociative Disorders: DSM-V and Beyond* (pp. 83–92). New York: Taylor & Francis Group.

English, D. J., et al. (2005) Defining Maltreatment Chronicity: Are There Differences in Child Outcomes? *Child Abuse and Neglect: The International Journal*, 29, pp. 575–595. DOI:10.1016/j.chiabu.2004.08.009.

ESTD (2017) Child and Adolescent Committee of the European Society on Trauma and Dissociation (ESTD). *Guidelines for the Assessment and Treatment of Children and Adolescents With Dissociative Symptoms and Dissociative Disorders*. Available at: www.estd.org (Accessed: 6 April 2021).

Freyd, J. (1996) *Betrayal Trauma: The Logic of Forgetting Childhood Abuse*. Cambridge: Harvard University Press.

Gil, E. (1991) *The Healing Power of Play: Working With Abused Children*. New York: Guilford Press.

Gomez, A. M. (2013) *EMDR Therapy and Adjunct Approaches With Children: Complex Trauma, Attachment, and Dissociation*. New York: Springer Publishing Company.

Herman, J. L. (1992) *Trauma and Recovery*. New York: Basic Books.

International Society for the Study of Trauma and Dissociation (ISSTD). (2003) Task Force on Children and Adolescents. *Guidelines for the Evaluation and Treatment of Dissociative Symptoms in Children and Adolescents*. Available at: www.isst-d.org (Accessed: 6 April 2021).

James, B. (1989) *Treating Traumatized Children: New Insights and Creative Interventions*. Lexington, MA: Lexington Books.

Kagan, R. (2014) Rebuilding Attachments With Traumatized Children: Healing from Losses, Violence, Abuse, and Neglect. New York: Taylor & Francis.

Kisiel, C., Stolbach, B. & Silberg, J. (2013) *Understanding and Addressing Dissociation Within Child Serving Systems: A Missing Link?* Philadelphia, PA: National Child Traumatic Stress Network All-Network Conference.

Landreth, G. L. (2012) *Play Therapy: The Art of the Relationship* (3rd ed.). New York: Routledge.

Linehan, M. M. (1993) *Skills Training Manual for Treating Borderline Personality Disorder*. New York: Guildford Press.

Liotti, G. (1999a) Disorganization of Attachment as a Model for Understanding Dissociative Pathology. In: Solomon, J. & George, C. (eds.) *Attachment Disorganization*. New York: Guilford Press.

Liotti, G. (1999b) Understanding the Dissociative Processes: The Contribution of Attachment Theory. *Psychoanalytic Inquiry*, 19(5), pp. 757–783.

Lowenstein, L. (2014) *Tips for Addressing Dissociation in Child and Play Therapy*. Available at: http://lianalowenstein.com/artProfDissociation.pdf (Accessed: 6 June 2021).

Mann, B. J. & Sanders, S. (1994) Child Dissociation and the Family Context. *Journal of Abnormal Child Psychology*, 22, pp. 373–388.

Myrick, A. C. & Green, E. J. (2014) Establishing Safety and Stabilization in Traumatized Youth: Clinical Implications for Play Therapists. *International Journal of Play Therapy*, 23(2), pp. 100–113. DOI: 10.1037/a0036397.

NCTSN. (2007) *Complex Trauma*. Available at: www.nctsn.org/trauma-types/complex-trauma (Accessed: 9 June 2021).

Ogawa, J., et al. (1997) Development and the Fragmented Self: Longitudinal Study of Dissociative Symptomatology in a Nonclinical Sample. *Development and Psychopathology*, 9(1), pp. 855–879.

Perry, B. D. (2001) The Neurodevelopmental Impact of Violence in Childhood. In: Schetky, D. & Benedek, E. P. (eds.) *Textbook of Child and Adolescent Forensic Psychiatry* (pp. 221–238). Washington, DC: American Psychiatric Press.

Perry, B. D. (2006) The Neurosequential Model of Therapeutics: Applying Principles of Neuroscience to Clinical Work With Traumatized and Maltreated Children. In: N. Boyd Webb (ed.) *Working With Traumatized Youth in Child Welfare* (pp. 27–52). New York: Guilford Press.

Perry, B. D. (2011) *Born for Love: Why Empathy Is Essential – and Endangered.* New York and Enfield: Harper Paperbacks; Publishers Group UK.

Perry, B. D. (2017) *The Boy Who Was Raised as a Dog: And Other Stories From a Child Psychiatrist's Notebook: What Traumatized Children Can Teach Us About Loss, Love, and Healing* (3rd ed.). New York: Basic Books.

Porges, S. (2011) *The Polyvagal Theory: Neurophysiological Foundations of Emotions, Attachment, Communication and Self-Regulation.* New York: W. W. Norton & Company.

Potgieter-Marks, R. (2012) When the Sleeping Tiger Roars – Perpetrator Introjects in Children. In: Vogt, R. (ed.) *Perpetrator Introjects – Psychotherapeutic Diagnostics and Treatment Models* (pp. 87–110). Kronig: Ansanger Verlag.

Putnam, F. W. (1989) *Diagnosis and Treatment of Multiple Personality Disorder.* New York: Guilford Press.

Rogers, C. (1951) *Client-Centered Therapy: Its Current Practice, Implications and Theory.* London: Constable.

Silberg, J. L. (2013) *The Child Survivor: Healing Developmental Trauma and Dissociation.* New York: Routledge.

Silberg, J. L. (2017) Trauma-Relevant Treatment of Dissociation for Children and Adolescents. In: Gold, S. N. (ed.) *APA Handbook of Trauma Psychology: Trauma Practice.* Washington, DC: American Psychological Association.

Silberg, J. L. & Dallam, S. (2010) Dissociation in Children and Adolescents: At the Crossroads. In: Dell, P. F. & O'Neil, J. A. (eds.) *Dissociation and Dissociative Disorders: DSM-V and Beyond.* Abingdon: Taylor and Francis Group.

Triplett, V. B. (2007) "Don't Talk!": Trauma and Dissociation in Play Therapy. In: Dugger, S. M. & Carlson, L. (eds.) *Critical Incidents in Counselling Children.* Alexandria, VA: American Counselling Association.

Van Der Kolk, B. (1987) *Psychological Trauma.* Washington, DC: American Psychiatric Publishing, Inc.

Van Der Kolk, B. (2014) *The Body Keeps the Score: Mind, Brain and Body in the Transformation of Trauma.* London: Penguin.

Waters, F. S. (2016) *Healing the Fractured Child.* New York: Springer.

Wieland, S. (ed.) (2015) *Dissociation in Traumatized Children and Adolescents Theory and Clinical Interventions* (2nd ed.). Hove: Taylor and Francis.

# Chapter 7

# I see you, you see me

## The personal process of a play therapy clinical supervisor

*Simon Kerr-Edwards*

As clinical supervisors, we hold up a mirror for the supervisee in order for them to reflect on their professional self and practice; to see, hear, critique and appreciate themselves and, through the development of the relationship, an ability to create a more effective and accurate picture of what it is they experience and achieve as practitioners. However, the mirror we hold is silvered by an understanding of our personal and professional self and therefore can both knowingly and unknowingly reflect our own process back to our supervisee. The angle at which the mirror is held by the supervisor may convey both the personal and professional concerns of the supervisor, highlighting to the supervisee the supervisor's own thoughts, feelings and preoccupations. In this chapter I am going to argue that the clinical supervisor needs to be cognisant of their own journey towards the person they are; their professional journey, their progression to becoming a clinical supervisor and how their experiences have become entwined to emerge as the supervisor-self that is seen by the supervisee. As with many interpersonal processes, being aware of what we consciously wish to show to others of our self and a preparedness to explore what we unconsciously reveal are vital to the ongoing development of personal awareness.

In beginning any heuristic self-examination, it is necessary to proceed with caution, as to understand one's own process as a clinical supervisor requires a combination of recollection, uncertainty and speculation in attempting to make connections across a considerable span of time and experience. Some of these links may be pertinent to the supervisor-self I now present and some may not, yet they illustrate the reflective nature of my journey and show my thinking as a supervisor. My ultimate aim is to not let this process obscure the supervisee's ability to see themselves in a helpful and congruent way. Being a role model for the supervisee is part of the dynamic of supervision but I also need to be aware that too strong a role model may inhibit their professional development and their ability to develop their own sense of themselves as a practitioner, or as Casement puts it, they may be "seriously undermined . . . feeling as if treatment (or even the patient) has been taken over by the supervisor" (1985: 24). Supervisors may tread a fine line in seeking to be clear and coherent in how they come across to their supervisee, whilst not wanting to stifle their ability to process and formulate what it is they are struggling with.

DOI: 10.4324/9781003017271-7

In principle, I want my supervisee to be congruent and authentic with me and I with them, in order for them to avoid saying what they think I want to hear and express themselves without caution. This is essential for me to gain a secure grasp of what is going on in their clinical work and therefore allow an exploration of their practice in its entirety. I want them to experience an authenticity of self from me whilst I bring forward, where appropriate, pertinent facets of my supervisor-self that can support their development. This may well involve making choices around what I say or show and possibly withholding those parts of myself that I deem unhelpful to them. In order for these choices to become a conscious decision, and not taken solely from habit, I need to combine a solid understanding of the developmental processes of the emerging play therapist along with an examination of the exclusive experiences and influences relevant to me personally.

For the play therapist, Le Vay explores the idea of being congruent and authentic as "recognising and accepting who we are, the individual and unique set of qualities, traits and characteristics that make up our self and how these become manifest within the relationship with the child" (2016: 4) and this is largely true of the supervisory relationship too. However, the supervisor must be mindful not to confuse their role with that of a therapist whilst acknowledging that the process can indeed be therapeutic. Confusing the supervisee as to the nature of the relationship needs avoiding and that examining their professional growth and development is not a replacement for their own personal therapy. The supervisor also needs to show that they are not a peer with the supervisee in the relationship and expect to be seen as a more experienced figure with whom they can allow themselves to be vulnerable, knowing that the supervisor will not match this vulnerability with their own. But as supervisor, we bring an understanding and awareness of our own vulnerability and a deep sense that we are familiar with these feelings (as we sit with them in our own clinical supervision) and knowledge that the process of being congruent and authentic with another can bring fear of exposure or shame. For all practitioners, this process of congruence and authenticity is especially challenging as we are often faced with children who are also in search of their congruent and authentic self, parents who may have lost their own ability to respond to their child with compassion, and professionals who are given limited time and resources to respond to their clients in a generous manner.

For the purpose of this chapter I will explore literature that highlights the supervisor's use of self and what this brings to the relationship. Then I will look at some personal and professional examples from my own supervisory experience (from the perspective of both supervisee and supervisor) and reflect on how these experiences influence my current supervisor-self.

## Understanding a supervisor's use of self

The therapeutic use of self by a therapist, its benefits and pitfalls, is well documented by Wosket (1999) and Baldwin (2013) and issues that arise from the use of self can equally be brought and explored within the supervision process. These discussions become crucial because as Kramer says

> [W]e are models, whether we like it or not. We can't help it. Whatever we are, we are. Those who spend time with us will make what they will of what they see and hear. Simply being in the same space, we present a style of being that may or may not be emulated.
>
> (2013: 37)

The same is true for the supervisor-supervisee dyad and as in therapy, the use of self by the supervisor contributes to this discussion. Knight (2012) encourages the supervisor to consider how they use their sense of self in supervision and to explore this issue with their supervisee as a means of getting them to reflect on their practice with clients and notes that "the supervisor's transparency can foster the supervisory alliance and lead to an environment in which the supervisee is more likely to be open and honest" (2012: 14). However, Knight adds that this needs to be carefully considered in order to avoid supervision becoming a therapy relationship, as highlighted earlier. McTighe (2011) supports the idea of the supervisor being a role model for the supervisee and interestingly, Gizynski (1978) suggests that this modelling can be more beneficial to the supervisee than just instruction on its own. Supervision approaches such as Hawkins and Shohet's (2012) Seven-Eyed Model incorporate the idea that the relationship between supervisee and supervisor is part of the process of supervision, that what happens between them may elicit some insight into the client-supervisee interactions or the supervisee's own process. This is developed in the work of Searles (2018) and his identification of a parallel process within supervision and, further to this, the exploring of countertransference in the supervisory relationship is encouraged by Strean (2005) who believes

> The supervisor's disclosure of her countertransference tends to make her appear much less authoritarian, more egalitarian, less of a wise expert and more of an authentic human being. This humane attitude of the supervisor helps reduce the supervisee's self-consciousness and need to appear omniscient.
>
> (Strean, 2005: 747)

Furthermore, Mothersole identifies three types of parallel process in supervision, with type three highlighting the dangers of "unresolved therapy issues, blind spots and skills deficits of the supervisor entering the process destructively" (1999: 118). This stresses the need for supervisors to be self-reflective and aware of their personal therapeutic and supervision journey and therefore ameliorate any potential negative impact within the supervision process.

One way the supervisor can overtly express their own processes to their supervisee is through the form of self-disclosure. Knox et al. (2008) highlight the advantages and disadvantages of self-disclosure and identify that this often happens when the supervisee was perceived as struggling by the supervisor. Furthermore, Farber identifies two particular patterns of disclosure by the supervisor, those that "spoke to the supervisors own experiences of clinical work; and those that took the form of emotionally resonant, empathic disclosures" (2006: 196). However, there are some words of caution about self-disclosure by the supervisor. As Page & Wosket say:

> Supervisors should be aware of suggesting, through self-disclosure about their own practice, something that the supervisee is not yet sufficiently skilled or experienced to do. This will at best confuse the supervisee, it may also leave them feeling incompetent. At worst, they may take a guess at what the supervisor means and then take a flying leap into the unknown by foisting this guesswork on the client.
>
> (2015: 111)

There are suggestions that those beginning their process of becoming supervisors reflect on their own professional journey and how they got to where they are now (Henderson et al. 2014) and for ongoing supervisors to keep reflecting on their journey and record their "philosophy of supervision" (Carroll, 2014: 190) or what supervision means to them in particular. Shohet and Shohet discuss the examining of core beliefs by the trainee supervisor; "beliefs about supervision, work, their culture, their society, their world and themselves" (2020: 59), adding that "it is not the beliefs . . . that cause problems . . . but the strength of our attachment and blindness to them" (2020: 59). This suggests that understanding the origin of our beliefs may enable supervisors to better monitor the impact of them in their work. For more personal reflections on their journey to becoming supervisors, Wilmot (2008) acknowledges the supervisory moments from her childhood as the early indications of the kind of supervisor that she would become and Carroll (2014) shares with us his personal influences as a supervisor and explores his personal struggle between reason and emotion and how this shaped his practice. Hewson and Carroll (2016) also talk about their journeys to becoming supervisors – how it took time to achieve a reflective supervisory position and how these insights shaped both themselves and in turn how they are seen by others.

## Personal supervisory experiences

My curiosity in exploring personal process begins with some trepidation, as identifying personal experiences which are connected to my self-as-supervisor may expose some vulnerability, but I contend that illuminating this journey can in turn positively benefit my supervisory practice and in turn my supervisees and their clients.

To begin with, I believe the primacy of *relationship* is rooted deeply within me, from having consistent and benign parental figures in my early life and being the youngest of three siblings in my birth family. I found myself surrounded by others and was soon drawn to the role of the observer, looking up and noticing relationships around me. This was a time of much playfulness and competition with humour as an interpersonal way of bonding. Little details and differences between myself and my family members both irritated and fascinated me, and my expression of feelings often led to me being seen as "overly sensitive" by them. Today I am able to tease them by saying I have made an entire career out of this sensitivity, but what I appreciate is that from this I developed a lack of sentimentality. My sister, two years older than myself, was my first "collegiate" and playful supervisor, someone who had my interest and welfare at heart, especially during the many times we played with other groups of children when adults were not around. Her regular presence allowed me to feel confident and take appropriate risks and she was also able to give me feedback, good and bad. As a secondary school and undergraduate student, although I had a wish to belong, my observer role remained strong and I was fascinated by, yet apart from, others and this led me to feel ambivalent towards belonging to groups, later identifying with Groucho Marx when he said "I don't want to belong to any club that will accept people like me as a member" (2009: 239). This lack of belonging also emerged as an oppositional streak, in part fuelled by feelings following the early death of my father and a general sensitivity to injustice and oppression. I wanted engagement with others but soon craved distance from them, a space from which I was able to examine or critique what I was part of. A student friend of the time said how they noticed that in group assignments, I would sit back and listen and allow others time to flail about and argue before becoming involved proposing solutions that synthesised the ideas that were being struggled with. Maybe this holding back and waiting stance is now a valuable supervisor-self trait for me. As an adult, becoming a parent was a pivotal point in my life, taking on the responsibility of nurturing and developing of small children and finding the right balance between boundaries and freedom as they developed and grew.

### Becoming a clinical supervisor

In hindsight, my journey to being a therapist seemed a coherent way of developing my curiosity for others and managing my sensitivity in a beneficial and productive way. However, the idea of becoming a clinical supervisor was not a role that occurred to me and the best way to describe it was that I "fell" into the role, as if it were a body of water, almost as soon as I qualified as a dramatherapist, firstly in my place of work and soon afterwards for dramatherapy students. However, I am a good swimmer, both literally and metaphorically. To imply I had no training would be wrong as I did attend some supervision courses and some of the ideas gained from them I still use today. What I remember of them is being drawn towards the facilitation of the learning process of others and focusing on them putting what we were being taught into practice. Remember, this was the mid-1980s, and clinical supervision was not yet established as an essential component of therapeutic practice and happily, today, there are clearer guidelines about this with opportunities to train and reflect on becoming a clinical supervisor.

## Examples from my clinical supervision experience

Since qualifying as a play therapist, I have had a number of supervisors, dozens of supervisees, both students and qualified, triads and groups, and from these experiences I would like to pick out some pivotal moments that have remained memorable for me and examine how they have reflected my development, impacted or challenged my practice and added the unique *silvering* to my supervisor mirror.

To illustrate my journey, I will focus on four examples from my clinical supervision, two from each side of the supervisory relationship and my experience both as supervisee and supervisor. These experiences continue to resonate with me as I write them and highlight my struggles from both sides of the relationship and just how powerful and challenging the experience of clinical supervision is. For these examples I have changed some details in order to protect the identity of those to whom I refer.

## Example one: starting out on my therapist journey

There is nothing more revealing than starting at the beginning with what was my first clinical supervision experience, as these first encounters can see the emergence of issues that might well be encountered further on in time. This small group experience was during my first placement as a dramatherapy student and I carried with me a combination of protective arrogance and reluctance to surrender to the process of being a student, a stressful time balancing the part-time course with a full-time job. My main preoccupation in the group was around being given direction by the supervisor on what I should be doing, and I became frustrated and disillusioned when I did not believe I was getting what I needed. Although unable to articulate this to the group at the time, I believe I wanted to be told what to do and I can now see that this conflicted with my supervisor who wanted me to explore, articulate or identify for myself what it was I needed to know. They were pressing me to do the reflective work when I wanted them to do it for me, and I personally experienced, or interpreted, this impasse as me not being good enough.

As a result, I wonder if we became caught up in a self-perpetuating loop; I pressed for something from them and they wanted something from me. On reflection, I see the paradox in my approach to this supervision; that I thought my supervisor was blocking my reflective capacity when it was more likely my anxiety that was restraining me. Feeling out of my depth as a student, I found it hard to accept the vulnerability of this position, or to own up to it to my supervisor. The group process possibly exacerbated this as what I saw reflected back to me were others in a very similar position, struggling to articulate the chaos of beginning a therapeutic journey, which I perceived as a joint despair at not getting what we wanted. This was a challenging experience for me but over the duration of the course, and especially through our student process group, I became more comfortable with balancing the need to reveal my struggle alongside the containment of my anxiety.

## Example two: inspiring and passionate supervision

My second example of being a supervisee is 15 years later, when I was a newly qualified play therapist and employed with a local authority that was embedded within the local child and adolescent mental health service. The post involved working with what was then termed looked-after children, now known as children-in-care, and children who had been adopted and I needed a clinical supervisor to support me. For this, I approached an experienced play therapist and supervisor who seemed a logical choice as I had consulted with them on other occasions in a previous work role and they had extensive experience with the client group. Our supervisory relationship lasted two years and was a memorable, influential experience that continues to inform my current practice.

In summary, I owe an enormous debt of gratitude for this experience of clinical supervision, which was a formative, grounding and at times exhilarating process. Our sessions were discursive and wide-reaching, with my supervisor having a tremendous turn of phrase, both witty and sharp-tongued. They spoke passionately about play therapy and in particular the rights of the child within the therapeutic process and I was in awe of their knowledge and wisdom and what I was able to learn from this experience. My supervisor promoted the principle of agency for the child who, when in the care system, often had little autonomy and control over decisions that impacted upon their lives. This ignited my passion for putting children at the heart of the therapeutic process and my supervisor challenged me to fit my therapeutic approach around the needs of the child and not vice versa, encouraging me to be creative in my thinking. Our conversations enabled me to formulate what I saw as the core principles of my clinical work and I felt endorsed and supported in doing this. I came out of sessions feeling energised and intellectually stimulated.

However, it is with some shame that I admit to also having struggled with aspects of our supervisory relationship. Inspiring as it was, I found it difficult to find my voice and develop my capacity for self-reflection within the relationship. My experience was that when I proposed a question or challenge that I was facing, my supervisor would start to expound their thoughts and analysis, which was challenging, thoughtful and wide-ranging and ultimately helpful. This didactic learning was exceptional, and I would listen and feel privileged to be getting such focused attention. But I do not remember much exploration of my own personal and professional process and I became content to be passive, sit back and listen (something I have already stated I am comfortable with) and to not engage too much with the supervisory conversation. On reflection, I see how I hid within my safe, default position as a learner, promoting my supervisor to the role of teacher and expert, which protected me from making myself vulnerable and risking the voicing of my thoughts and feelings. By not speaking out my internal process I was protecting myself from being seen as getting it wrong which, as a newly qualified play therapist was maybe too unsettling for me, especially as I already saw myself as an experienced professional. There seemed an ironic parallel process at play here, between losing my own therapist voice whilst advocating for the voice of the child.

## Example three: my supervisor journey begins

This is an example from my own early experience of supervising that highlights the need to emotionally contain what is presented to us. Concurrent with the time of my dramatherapy training, I was employed by a residential community for 16–21-year-olds with complex needs, and as part of a new role within the organisation, I took on the supervision of several residential workers. Having been through the care system, the young people we were working with had never established any stability in their lives due to chaotic and traumatic childhoods, and subsequently they were unused to adults who were reliable and benign. The challenging nature of the work was explored by the organisation through a regular individual and group supervisory framework that focused on the interpersonal and relational challenges to the work and where supervisees were expected to explore how the work impacted on their sense of self.

My first supervisee was a colleague who I thought of as having a good mix of robust and sensitive qualities with excellent relationships with the young people. At the time of our first meeting, they arrived ashen-faced and seemed totally at a loss when they sat down. I asked what the matter was, and they told me they had just received a call from the hospital to say that they had skin cancer. This was an unforgettable moment and still, nearly 35 years later, I experience a physiological reaction to the memory as I write these words. Unsurprisingly, my supervisee was devastated and distraught and we stayed with this for a few minutes, still taking in the news together. I recall saying something like "take this one step at a time", "this is treatable" and "it sounds as if they have detected this in a timely manner", but my words in that moment seemed strange and unwieldy. I soon sent them home to get support from their family.

This moment stays with me for a number of reasons, some personal and some professional. As referred to earlier, I had lost my own father to cancer so I had experienced the devastating and uncertain challenge that living with a cancer diagnosis can be. But I balanced this with the belief that despite the loss of a parent I had carried on, still able to function and then emotionally re-group, so facing and exploring existential issues of living and dying was something I was familiar with. My instinct at the time was to focus on emotionally holding my supervisee as they needed time to gain personal support and seek swift treatment but I soon shared some of my personal process as a means of opening up a dialogue between us. The diagnosis became the focus of the sessions over the following weeks and over the next year of our relationship, we moved beyond the shock into learning

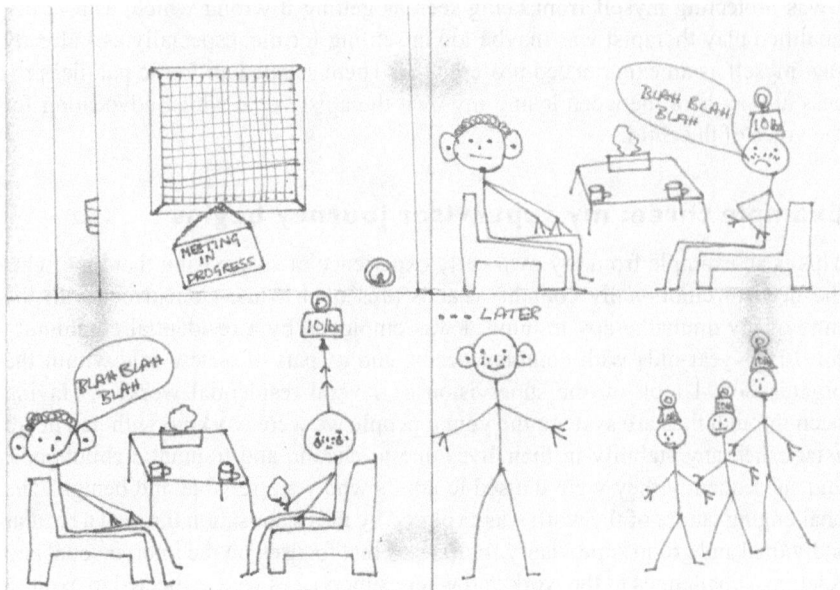

*Figure 7.1* Represents our supervision journey together and is a graphic portrayal of the benefit of supervision

to live with uncertainty, although the prognosis for recovery was good. Figure 7.1 illustrates our supervision journey together and was, a while later, my leaving present from my supervisee. Unsurprisingly (for those who know me), I am represented by the figure with the curly hair and my supervisee with the freckles. I have big ears and am listening to them talk. As we talk, the weight upon my supervisee's head is lifted and in turn they are able to grow ears like mine as they support the young people, who themselves are weighed down. This is a simple but graphic portrayal of the benefit of supervision.

But supervision is made up of a number of functions, and I was keen to concentrate our conversation on developing their therapeutic skills with the clients whilst still being attentive to their health struggle. But I found it hard to sustain this focus as the shadow of cancer was a continuing backdrop to our dialogue and we would often return to the subject. But I have often wondered whether the fact my supervisee's health issue arising at the beginning of our relationship might have inhibited me, making it harder to move the dialogue into other more challenging areas.

## Example four: supervisor dilemma

Considerations of the appropriateness and longevity of therapeutic work are common in clinical supervision and through the following example, I will highlight how constant questioning and self-doubt is part of this process for the supervisor. This example is of my supervision of an experienced play therapist who was a warm, empathic and capable independent practitioner who managed their own caseload of children with complex trauma histories. Our relationship was mutually respectful, and I perceived them as thoughtful, questioning and welcoming of what I had to offer. They would consult me on formulating treatment plans and shared with me the emotional impact of the work. Our relationship lasted several years and during this time, there was one particular client who became a challenge for us both and who, within supervision, became a frequent source of discussion. The client's presentation appeared relatively straightforward to begin with but soon became more challenging as issues emerged about the safety of both the client and my supervisee. Initially, we discussed about what might be put in place to manage these safety concerns, how the client could be supported outside of sessions and how the supervisee might establish effective boundaries within the sessions. This led to a small reduction in our anxiety, but progress remained slow and patchy and after a while this led me to propose to my supervisee the idea that they refer the client elsewhere. My suggestion was met with resistance as my supervisee argued that they were too deep into the therapeutic process to withdraw and how termination at this stage could itself be unsafe and on reflection, I conceded their point. But this made me feel no better and I became increasingly anxious every time we discussed the client within supervision, leading me to feel overwhelmed by a situation that I had little or no control over. I was not in the room with the client so had no experience of them other than through what was presented within supervision, but what I heard left me continuing to doubt the appropriateness of the work, placing me in a conflicted position. During this time, I took these feelings of powerlessness to my own clinical supervision and similarly, our process became dominated by this client and the conflict I was experiencing. But my supervisor, whose judgement I trusted, helped me to contain my anxiety and enabled me to continue to support my supervisee. As time went on, the client gradually began to stabilise, and between us, the supervisee and I held together the work towards a successful conclusion.

## Further reflections on these experiences

The beginning of a journey can often reveal so much of what is to follow. Possibly, my first supervisory experience resonates more with me because I was at the start of something and had yet to grasp what was required of me. Here, I see myself struggling with what I needed; sensitive to evaluation, wanting certainty and guidance from my supervisor whilst being dismissive of the facilitative stance they took. My inability to articulate what I needed was blocking me from connecting with the process and now, on reflection, I can see how my supervisor wished me to explore my resistance, which I was not ready to do. A combination of my anxiety and the group process led to an experience that was at the time frustrating, but that now illuminates the sensitivity of the student's relationship with their supervisor.

The supervisor I am today would look to take a more didactic stance with a student, one that offers clear guidance and instruction, leaving less room for ambiguity and misunderstanding, a balance of acknowledging the anxiety with some direction as to how to proceed. I identify with Ray's (2011) *process of play therapy supervision* where she matches supervisee dynamics in supervision with responsive qualities of the clinical supervisor. At this early stage, the supervisor is encouraged to exhibit a significant amount of empathy for the supervisee along with instruction, in order to contain anxiety. The most likely inhibitor of self-reflection is anxiety and I would encourage all supervisors to pay attention to this when working with students as they grapple with putting newly acquired skills into practice.

My second example was from the period of my emerging and developing passion for play therapy and my supervisor was an inspiration and role model who I wished to emulate and, in time, live up to. The energetic display of their therapist identity connected with my drive to engage with young people in order to deliver a unique and transformative experience. At this time, my core principles of good practice were still being forged and when I express these ideas with my supervisees some 20 years later, I can still connect with the passionate voice of my supervisor of that time. Their apparent fearlessness impressed me and their wish to come up against and re-examine common theory chimes with an oppositional streak in me. I cannot be as fearless as they when my self-doubt encroaches, but I advocate the idea that, as therapists, we must not be afraid to say the unsayable or avoid what is uncomfortable.

The by-product of such a strong role model was that I found myself unable to find my voice or develop the self-reflective qualities that I now see I lacked at that time. As a newly emerging play therapist I had much more experience of the therapeutic process than I did during my training but I still found it hard to insert myself into the process. I was quite happy to sit back and enjoy the experience rather than try and forge my own identity as distinct from that of my supervisor. This is a central dilemma I now experience as a supervisor: when to inspire others and share expertise and when to give space to allow the supervisee to grapple with and mould their own separate identity. Being explicit about what I think is a vital part of my process as a supervisor, but I have to be mindful that this might come across as telling my supervisee what to do and inhibit their ability to formulate ideas for themselves and, as Casement (1985) warns, I must not try to take over their process with mine. At the time I can see that I wanted to agree with and impress my supervisor but in doing so avoided engaging in my own learning process with all its doubts and mistakes.

A supervisor must, as must any therapist, be ready for the issues coming through the door, and my third example provided a powerful lesson in the value of emotional preparedness. Being attentive to the supervisee's preoccupations on arrival to supervision is required before the work of reflection can begin. Distractions of thought may need to be expressed and then put to one side in order for the supervisee to be in a place where they can focus on the task in hand. How easy or difficult it might be for the supervisee to "park" their preoccupations might need to be addressed, and the supervisor may be required to guide and support them in doing this. But my experience also points to how challenging the disclosure of the cancer diagnosis was so early in our relationship, before it had assumed a rhythm of trust and appreciation. Looking back, my concern is whether the disclosure led to us becoming locked into a therapeutic (rather than supervisory) relationship early on in the process and I question whether I was able to be more balanced in my work and able to shift the conversation when required. Did the powerful nature of facing life and death challenges hinder my ability to fully explore all aspects of my supervisee's therapeutic work? This also highlights a broader issue that still preoccupies me – how, once we have an established supervisory relationship, do we shift our patterns of conversations in order that we keep alert to the changing needs of the supervisee and their therapeutic work?

We all face personal challenges at different life stages; parenthood or non-parenthood, relationship breakdowns, financial or health concerns, responsibilities for ageing relatives, loss and bereavement, and these are all crucial in forming who we are and are influential in how we become therapists and supervisors. My early loss of a parent was an emotionally shaping moment, not something that I believe held me back but rather propelled me forward with a renewed vigour. However, I see that such personal challenges need to be held in perspective, alongside with the work done in supervision: work that holds the client's welfare at its heart. Here, as I did then, the use of self-disclosure may help as a means of putting personal challenges into perspective and modelling what it is we can do when these challenges become such as to affect our ability to carry out our work.

The inclusion of my fourth example is in the hope that it will resonate with other supervisors, as I believe it illustrates a common challenge for us as we try and enable our supervisees to plot a course of action through often complex and unpredictable work. Supervision is about working with what is reported to us, either through words, symbols or video, and we often do not have the full felt sense or understanding of how the work is progressing. Here, I became uncertain as to how much of my anxiety and concern to express back to my supervisee and how much to engage them in the emerging parallel process between us. I expressed some of my thoughts but contained the full extent of my anxiety and holding this position was uncomfortable, especially as I commonly aim to freely express myself as supervisor. The experience of self-doubt can be important as the therapeutic process is an inexact science and progress often emerges out of challenging and difficult moments. The tension of balancing both the welfare of my supervisee and their client led at times to an uncertain and anxious personal and professional process, of which I was cognisant but still uneasy.

A vital component of this process was that of my own supervision and the importance of being thoughtfully held by my supervisory relationship in order for me in turn to be able to hold the work of my supervisee. Having another voice, benign, trustworthy and challenging, that could help me express my dilemmas and formulate my thinking, enabled me to pass this back to my supervisee. Throughout this period of work, I was indebted to the skilful grace and determination shown by my supervisor in managing this sometimes bewildering process with me, and I continue to be so.

## Not forgetting . . .

Another thread that consistently runs through my supervisory experiences is my admiration for my supervisees at all levels of experience. I am consistently impressed by their conceptualisation skills, reflective ability and sheer persistence, qualities that make the role of clinical supervisor so rewarding. We all need validation for what we do, and supervisees may often be expecting criticism rather than a compliment or appreciation and so I seek to express my admiration when I experience it. On occasion I have thought "I couldn't have handled that as well as you did" or "I'm not sure I could have been creative in that situation" or even "you are a better play therapist than me". At times my admiration for the sophistication of their thinking, regardless of their experience, both humbles and spurs me on, without challenging my own sense of self-worth. My role is to facilitate their process and not compete for who is best and as Shohet and Shohet contend, "see all students as 'A' students" (2020: 29). In them I can also see the quality of teaching they have received and how this has improved over time, sometimes leaving me with a degree of envy. I want to record here just how much I, as a supervisor, learn from my supervisees and if you as a supervisor are not learning something from your supervisee, then you are missing a big opportunity and a valuable part of the process.

A striking theme within these reflections is the potential for disconnect between supervisor and supervisee and how the tension between "wanting and giving" can lead to challenges in the relationship. As supervisees, articulating what it is we want or need may be difficult, as is the recognition of these signals by the supervisor. The responsibility to attend to this matching belongs mostly with the supervisor who may need to adapt their supervisor-self in order to meet the supervisee's need. But responsibility also lies with the supervisee who must strive to be coherent in what it is they are looking for or needing from their supervisor. A regular conversation about how the supervisory relationship is meeting the needs of the supervisee, and ultimately the clients, is a necessary part of the relationship and must not be avoided. In order to do this, I recommend that supervision be a place for both seriousness and playfulness, an arena wherein both supervisor and supervisee can creatively explore the profundities of the powerful therapeutic work and their respective core beliefs in order to avoid the traps of certainties and absolutes and also laugh at one's own patterns, tendencies and mistakes as wonderful byproducts of the journey. Carroll's "Bullshit Detector" (2014: 184) provides the spirited voice of a kindred supervisor.

Putting this chapter together has been an enlightening and sometimes challenging process and highlights how we as clinical supervisors are shaped by our personal and professional experiences in order to become the supervisors we are. My hope has been to demonstrate how reflection upon my personal process is a means of examining the supervisor-self seen by my supervisees. The journey of a clinical supervisor can often be complex and unpredictable and in my experience, congruence and authenticity are the most important factors that contribute towards successful outcomes, as well as a comprehensive understanding of one's own process of becoming and being a supervisor. Alongside this is an ability to be flexible and thoughtful in how we present to our supervisees, creating a relationship that is both unique and meaningful. Supervision is relational and intersubjective and in this sense the acknowledgement of each other's personal and professional process is a significant contributory factor in the development of a successful supervisory relationship.

## References

Baldwin, M. (ed.) (2013) *The Use of Self in Therapy* (3rd ed.). Hove: Routledge.

Carroll, M. (2014) *Effective Supervision for the Helping Professions* (2nd ed.). London: Sage.

Casement, P. (1985) *On Learning from the Patient*. London: Tavistock.

Farber, B. (2006) *Self-Disclosure in Psychotherapy*. New York: Guildford Press.

Gizynski, M. (1978) Self Awareness of the Supervisor in Supervision. *Clinical Social Work Journal*, 6(3), pp. 202–210.

Hawkins, P. & Shohet, R. (2012) *Supervision in the Helping Professions* (4th ed.). Maidenhead: Open University Press.

Henderson, P., Holloway, J. & Miller, A. (2014) *Practical Supervision*. London: Jessica Kingsley.

Hewson, D. & Carroll, M. (2016) *Reflective Practice in Supervision*. Mossbrook: Hazelbrook.

Knight, C. (2012) Therapeutic Use of Self: Theoretical and Evidence-Based Considerations for Clinical Practice and Supervision. *The Clinical Supervisor*, 31, pp. 1–24.

Knox, S., Burkard, A. W., Edwards, L. M., Smith, J. J. & Schlosser, L. Z. (2008) Supervisors' Reports of the Effects of Supervisor Self-Disclosure on Supervisees. *Psychotherapy Research*, 18(5), pp. 543–549.

Kramer, C. H. (2013) Revealing Our Selves In: Baldwin, M. (ed.) *The Use of Self in Therapy* (3rd ed., pp. 36–63). Hove: Routledge, 2016.

Le Vay, D. (2016) To Be or Not to Be? In: Le Vay, D. & Cuschieri, E. (eds.) *Challenges in Theory and Practice of Play Therapy* (pp. 1–17). Abingdon: Routledge.

Marx, G. (2009) *Groucho and Me*. London: Virgin.

McTighe, J. P. (2011) Teaching the Use of Self Through the Process of Clinical Supervision. *Clinical Social Work Journal*, 39(3), pp. 301–307.

Mothersole, G. (1999) Parallel Process: A Review. *The Clinical Supervisor*, 18(2), pp. 107–121.

Page, S. & Wosket, V. (2015) *Supervising the Counsellor and Psychotherapist* (3rd ed.). Hove: Routledge.

Ray, D. C. (2011) *Advanced Play Therapy*. Abingdon: Routledge.

Searles, H. F. (2018) The Informational Value of the Supervisor's Emotional Experience. In: *Collected Papers on Schizophrenia and Related Subjects* (pp. 157–176). Abingdon: Routledge.

Shohet, R. & Shohet, J. (2020) *In Love With Supervision*. Monmouth: PCCS Books.

Strean, H. R. (2005) Resolving Therapeutic Impasses by Using the Supervisor's Countertransference. In: Turner, F. J. (ed.) *Social Work Diagnosis in Contemporary Practice* (pp. 739–749). Oxford: Oxford University Press.

Wilmot, J. (2008) The Supervisory Relationship: A Lifelong Calling. In: Shohet, R. (ed.) *Passionate Supervision* (pp. 88–109). London: Jessica Kingsley.

Wosket, V. (1999) *The Therapeutic Use of Self: Counselling Practice, Research and Supervision*. London: Routledge.

# Chapter 8

# The art*isans* of the relationship

## An exploration of trainee vulnerability

*Maria Victoria Aralde*

## Introduction

My play therapy training had an immense impact on me. When asked in my interview if I was ready for the demands of the training, I confidently replied "yes" along with a list of reasons why. However, soon after starting the training I realised the little I knew about what the real demands of the training would be, finding myself immersed in a highly emotional and personal journey, an aspect of the process that I had clearly underestimated.

During the training, I felt drawn to a space of vulnerability where I faced uncertainty and anxiety, and many times wondered if I would be able to complete the programme. I regularly heard the phrase "trust the process", however the process seemed overwhelming at times. It was not an easy or comfortable encounter but it was part of the journey into self-reflection. In order to relate in an empathetic manner and empower the child, it is essential that we, therapists, are able to embrace our vulnerability. This in turn helps us to recognise both our shared humanity and our right to not be perfect, and is what enables our self-acceptance. As Brown (2015) suggests, vulnerability is the core, the heart, the centre of meaningful human experiences.

I believe this chapter could be read as a cautionary tale for students who are beginning this journey. Perhaps this narrative could also be felt as a "hand on the shoulder" when feeling overwhelmed, and at the same time it might work as a reminder to *trust the process*.

The play therapy MA programme at the University of Roehampton is based on the person-centred perspective of psychotherapy developed by Carl Rogers (2003). This approach emphasises a movement away from the psychoanalytic tradition of interpretation and diagnosis towards a more active listening to the client's process. Rogers' hypothesis was that the client is the one who knows what hurts and has an instinctive direction towards healing. He conceptualised "actualisation" as the constitutive, motivational and constructively directional tendency towards growth and fulfilment. He also argued that the sense of being "human" is organised in the relational space with another, hence individual experiences become influenced in terms of the positive regard of the "significant other" and in

DOI: 10.4324/9781003017271-8

this scenario, the individual begins to discriminate their experiences according to "conditions of approval" (Rogers, 2003: 498).

Grounded in Roger's work, Axline (2002) developed a new therapeutic approach for working with children: non-directive play therapy. In addition, Landreth (2012) and Moustakas (2007, 1990), amongst others, are of important influence in the play therapy field, highlighting the relational dimension of the child-centred approach. Thus, child-centred play therapy (CCPT) is based upon the relationship between the child and the therapist and is rooted in the therapist's total acceptance of the child. By feeling fully accepted, the child is free to explore and make sense of different life experiences. In this context, the personhood of the therapist is an important element within the therapeutic relationship, and this signifies the importance of therapeutic presence as the foundation for empathy, unconditional positive regard and congruence, which were defined by Rogers as the core conditions for a healing therapeutic relationship (Rogers, 2003).

The concept of self-awareness within the therapist is of great importance. It alludes to the capacity to know oneself; one's own internal experiences and consequent reactions and is a basis for the therapeutic work. Therapists should be aware of the distinction between personal feelings and those that might arise within the context of the therapeutic relationship as this is a crucial element for the practice of congruence, genuineness, transparency and empathy. Underpinned by these core conditions, the relationship between therapist and client is based on trust, that is that both therapist and client are trustworthy.

Blanco et al. (2014) point out that the tradition of therapeutic training programs often seems to be focused primarily on the development of skills and techniques, perhaps because the teaching of technical skills is less complex than enhancing the self-awareness of the trainee. Similarly, Aguilera (2009), in her study of developmental experiences of newly qualified play therapists, argues that "there are other aspects to learning, such as emotions, personal needs, developing confidence, and evaluating self" (Aguilera, 2009: 212). Aguilera's statement seems to highlight a model of training that does not prioritise the emotional involvement of the self of the trainee, which I would suggest is essential for the development of self-awareness. On the basis of this study, Aguilera recommends a holistic approach to CCPT training, including elements of self-care and the inclusion of personal therapy for trainees.

This kind of humanistic and holistic approach in training is a core component of the CCPT MA Programme at the University of Roehampton, which includes challenging students to be self-aware in order to become more attentive, connected and present within their therapeutic practice. Alongside the teaching of therapeutic skills, the training provides the flexibility for students to experience and explore feelings of conflict and self-doubt as a foundation for self-reflection, which in turn will help them become more fully present and accepting of the client.

Alongside the academic modules of the programme, trainees are involved in experiential activities that demand an emotional engagement with both others and themselves. These include personal therapy, experiential process group, infant observation, expression through creative media, placement and clinical supervision. The conceptualisation and delivery of the programme take the trainee to a space of self-reflection that, in my experience, was overwhelming at times; the interpersonal formation of a new identity facilitated through the development of self-awareness and a redefinition of past experiences.

## Trainee vulnerability

The Oxford Living Dictionary's (2017) definition of vulnerability is "the quality or state of being exposed to the possibility of being attacked or harmed, either physically or emotionally". In professional fields such as architecture, engineering and business, it is very common to consider or even measure the variable of vulnerability, for which potential levels of risk are assessed to prevent certain circumstances or events causing harm. In the personal field, Brown (2015) studied the experience of vulnerability in the general population (without a specific background) and she defined vulnerability as having the characteristics of uncertainty, risk and emotional exposure.

The vulnerability that I faced during the training felt like an emotional assault. Suddenly rather than gradually, I experienced a sense of losing control of my feelings and, ultimately, I was trying to keep hold of my grip whilst feeling that I was being pushed to the edge, juggling my emotions alongside the academic and everyday day demands of life. I felt lost and unsure of what I was doing. During group activities, a solitary space for reflection was activated, with the disturbing feeling of being extremely exposed. This feeling of exposure came from a sense of being in the spotlight, even when the one holding the light was myself, like being thrown into space without a spacesuit. I became angry with a process that felt contradictory – that in a non-judgemental space I was beginning to feel judged and uncontained.

As Rønnestad and Skovholt (2003) suggest, the emotional impact of personal and professional development can be intense, wherein trainees are required to reflect upon their personal past experiences, often in the context of a training group, which can engender feelings of exposure, comparison and judgement. Feeling vulnerable, I had the need to be recognised and validated as "good enough". The concept of being good enough has had a significant impact on me and was something I sought to internalise during my training journey. Furthermore, by being part of a wider culture that generally associates vulnerability with weakness, the reflexive nature of the training was, at the beginning, disturbing and overwhelming.

The different aspects of the self revealed through this process of experiential learning are well described within the conceptual model (Fig. 8.1) of the Johari Window (Luft & Ingham, 1955).

| Arena | Blind Spot |
|---------|------------|
| Façade | Unknown |

*Figure 8.1* The Johari Window (Luft & Ingham, 1955)

Within this model, the experience of self is categorised into four areas: The "arena" represents the known self that everyone can see; the "façade" corresponds to the self that we can see but it is unavailable or hidden to others; the "blind spot" consists of the self that others can see in us but we cannot and the "unknown" involves the area that neither us nor others know about.

Reflecting upon this model, my experience of vulnerability is located within complexity of the interactions of the four quadrants, between what is known and unknown to the self in a relational environment. In this context I was able to encounter aspects of myself that I was not completely aware of, experienced as an internal battle to hold myself in one piece. During the training, I vividly remember as never before my childhood, my troubled adolescence and how I felt at the time; confused, lost, lonely and in pain – looking for affection and a role model and making difficult choices. I came to understand the shame and blame that I felt, which only reinforced my confusion and lack of worthiness. I was able to connect with the adolescent that somehow was hurting herself in every sense, and I became quite sad about "that girl". As far away in time and distance that I was from that child, it all came up during training.

This connection of feelings from early childhood became especially prominent during my placement, when I became aware that I was finding it challenging to communicate with a parent of a child. The parent presented as emotionally unavailable for the child, and I felt frustrated by our struggle to communicate effectively as if we were speaking two different languages. Reflecting upon this process in my personal therapy and supervision helped me to understand this within the context of unconscious communication, and the parent's possible projection of feelings of inadequacy, as this was the way that I felt in relation to her. Alongside this were my own childhood feelings in relation to parent unavailability and my consequent identification with the child I was working with. I was aware of feeling preoccupied by feelings of abandonment and of "judging" or "taking the child's side" in relation to the parent. I was surprised and fearful of the strength of my feelings and the impact they were having on my capacity to establish a therapeutic channel of communication. Personal therapy helped me to identify and explore these feelings, and I was able to move from a place of over-identification to a position of feeling more grounded in my role of play therapist.

## Vulnerability within experiential process group

Experiential process group is a learning and therapeutic space that contributes to the development of self-awareness in trainees by providing the opportunity to reflect upon their personal process within the relational context of a group (Le Vay & Cuschieri, 2016).

The experience of process group brought another opportunity to look inward. In the journal that I kept during the training, I defined the experience of the process group as a "revolution", highlighting the two component words of "revolve" and "evolution" as an apt linguistic representation of the emotional demands involved in the process.

In the first stage of the group process, there seemed to be a strong need for unity. Having been brought together as participants within the shared, intimate space of the group, it was very disconcerting and upsetting at times to experience the distress of others, and I personally felt afraid of emotional collapse.

Feeling "part of" and "included" represented a strong aspect of the experience for me as I have been in and out of many groups during the course of my life. Some of those circumstances were not my choice – moving 800 km from where I used to live when I was 11 years old, moving between different schools throughout my adolescence. Other decisions, like moving to the United Kingdom during my adulthood, were my own. Still, my decision or not, these experiences reinforced the sense of either belonging or not belonging.

I believe that the common experience that we (the participants of the group) most identified with was the anxiety in relation to what we "should be doing". I personally needed some direction, someone to tell me what to do and if what we were doing was right or wrong. Upon reflection, I realised that I was unconsciously seeking approval/validation from the group facilitator, just as I did with my father.

My father left my house when I was 11 years old and it was an episode that had a significant impact upon my confidence. Reflecting on how those years felt, I came to understand that I lived for many years with the unconscious feeling that I was not worthy enough for my father "to stay", as if he had found something better. I remember that there was a character in a television show that I felt both attracted to and terrified of at the same time. It was the Incredible Hulk. Dr. Banner was a physician and scientist, traumatised by an accident that killed his beloved wife. During an experiment, Banner was bombarded with gamma radiation, which caused him to transform into the "Hulk" whenever he became overwhelmed by anger or distress. To keep from being discovered, Banner travels from town to town in search of a cure. I now think that I was identifying myself with that "monster" and was scared of letting go of the angry, chaotic feelings that I was experiencing for fear of losing control.

Conflict was an intrinsic part of the process group experience and evoked powerful memories of my broken family and how that felt as a child. I was in survival mode and, like my experience within the group, trying to make sense of a situation. My childhood house was for me a very sad place to be and could, to some extent, be compared to the "silence" of the group that at times felt unbearable. We were all (my family/the group) grieving for what we had lost; that our experience of conflict meant that things would never be the same. Furthermore, I was an active participant in the group conflict, attracting the label of troublemaker, just like my teenage days.

The experience of the group also provided the opportunity to reflect on my relationship with my siblings, due to the familiarity and intimacy of the familial context, recognising and sharing interests alongside the emotional intensity connected to this experience. These relationships (siblings/group participants) presented opportunities for emotional reciprocity that were sustaining and nurturing. But at other times, distressful and painful memories from the past were triggered and both within my sibling group and the process group we sometimes felt unknown to each other, shut down through a state of emotional disconnection.

## Vulnerability within infant observation

Alongside my experience of the process group, I was also engaged in a process of infant observation that drew my attention to the evolution of family relationships and the early developmental processes involved in a newly configured family. A total of 30 weekly one-hour observations allowed me to identify unconscious aspects of behaviour, patterns of communication, moments of rupture and repair and the development of relationships within the dynamic interaction of the family. The different perspectives of the observer's role and the emotional impact of the experience were important and personally significant aspects of the experience. As in other elements of the training, the process of infant observation requires the capacity to manage often very anxious feelings and, in this context, those feelings that can arise in response to the demands of a new-born baby.

Initially, I found the role of observer challenging and found myself feeling emotionally overwhelmed as I intruded into this private family space. This was the mother's second child and in the context of emotional vulnerability, I began to think about the mother feeling fragmented by the demands of her two children. I speculated about the newborn baby becoming a priority for the mother, in terms of its innate defenselessness and the maternal preoccupation demanded in providing for the infant's needs. I wondered about the older child that has to wait and the subsequent feelings of guilt that might arise in the mother. I also felt guilty as an observer; I too was prioritising the baby. The arrival of a sibling is a deprivation for the elder child, a loss that can be expressed in different ways, perhaps in the form of destructive envy or defiance towards the parents. Over the course of the observations, I was at times the one who paid most attention to the elder child and I am aware that I allowed her to place me in that position, mostly because her demands were explicit and forceful but also because of my own, strong feelings of identification.

Once again, I was in an intimate space engaging in a truly meaningful relationship and once again, I was taken by surprise. For almost nine months I visited the family weekly and whilst maintaining the role of observer, our greetings became less rigid, our gaze conveyed a shared understanding and I felt more attuned to the mother's feelings. During the course of the observations, I drank many imaginary cups of tea and enjoyed the cupcakes that were offered to me. I embraced the new dimensions of the observations when the baby started to crawl and I became an object of exploration, starting with my shoes. I felt extremely touched when the mother held the two children and danced to one of her favourite songs. Inside, I too was dancing; I felt privileged and grateful to witness their time together.

Towards the end of the observations, I found out that I was expecting a baby and the process became even more moving, despite my emotional fragility. Unfortunately, the day before the final observation, I experienced a missed miscarriage and although this was deeply challenging and difficult personal experience, the meaningful relationships I had formed during the course of my training enabled me to explore my feelings of vulnerability from different perspectives.

### Notes from final infant observation

*Two days ago, I found out that my pregnancy ended in a missed miscarriage and although I was feeling physically and emotionally unwell, I decided to attend my observation to say goodbye. On arrival mother greets me at the door and tells me that she needs to take sister to the nursery and asks me if I would like to go. Sister looks at me and smiles looking at a couple of bags that I have in my hand. I smile at her and I give her a bag. She opens it and takes out a soft toy (monkey) and, smiling, thanks me. Baby is on the floor and he crawls towards me. I kneel and give him a bag. Sister moves close to help him and takes the monkey out of the bag. Baby holds the monkey with both hands and immediately places his mouth on the monkey's face. Sister comments that they both have the same monkey and I smile. She takes her monkey and makes it kiss Baby's monkey. Baby smiles and bounces up and down with excitement. I feel terribly emotional and I want to leave as soon as I can.*

*I give mother a present that I have for her. She asks if I am crazy and says that I shouldn't do that. She opens the bag with excitement and takes out the cookery book that is inside. She shouts with excitement and hugs me and says "before we start crying let's go to the car". We all leave the house and walk to the car. Sister and Baby sit in the back seat, both of them holding their monkeys, and I sit at the front with mother. She tells me that she will make one of the recipes from the book because Sunday is her birthday and surprised, I tell her that it is my child's birthday as well. We arrive at the nursery and I get out of the car to say goodbye to Sister. I wish her a great day at Nursery and hug her. I remain standing by the car looking at Baby as mother walks Sister to the entrance. She comes back and we drive back to the house.*

*On the way back I decided that I will not enter the house. We arrive and I tell mother that I am going to leave. She asks me if I am sure and whether I would like to have a coffee with her and I cannot hold back my tears. I tell her that I think that it is better to leave. Mother invites me to hold Baby and I do it without being able to stop my tears. Baby smiles at me and I smile back. Mother gives me a hug and I feel that I will fall apart and cannot talk. She asks me to visit her at some point and I reply that I will. She wishes me the best with my studies and I wish the best to her. I thank her and start walking away. Mother takes Baby's hand and waves at me. I wave back and walk to my car.*

This was not the ending that I wanted. Not for my pregnancy. Not for the observations. Not for the relationship with mother, baby and sister. They deserved more but I could not do it. I could not accept a coffee with mother in our last time together.

Group seminar sessions provided me with the opportunity to share and reflect upon my experience of the final observation. As my peers began talking about their own observations, I felt myself starting to emotionally collapse. I shared with the group my frustration, anger, blame and pain and I felt listened to, supported and contained and they encouraged me to arrange a visit to the family in order to experience a "good enough" ending. I was grateful to my peers that they could understand the deep personal significance and meaning of the observation experience and why I felt as I did in relation to the ending.

Vulnerability is a key element within this modality of training. However, this requires a level of self-awareness to be able to identify what belongs to whom within the therapeutic context. Our personal circumstances do influence our responses, but the use of effective self-awareness and reflective thinking helps us to remain connected with our experiences from a place where we can use ourselves in a more therapeutic manner.

After having a first meeting with a parent in placement I reflected on the emotional impact of that encounter. There was a moment when the parent was describing her feelings of anger and how lonely the process of grief was for her. At that moment, I could feel "in my bones" what the mother was expressing, and was triggered by my own experience of loss. It was my anger that I was feeling and I commented to the parent that I understood more than she might think. Although I believe that I acted with honesty and genuineness, I was aware at that moment that something was not right in terms of my therapeutic response. I reflected upon this with both my supervisor and therapist, and it was clear to me that I had spoken from my own needs, although the parent also shared that no one had spoken to her in that way before and that no-one understood how she was feeling. We went on to build an excellent therapeutic relationship although I recognised that my own personal feelings and responses were an active part of this process.

## Vulnerability and personal therapy

Personal therapy was an important part of my development, both personally and professionally, and it is an important element for the facilitation of self-awareness for trainees. It is the space that offers the opportunity to explore any unresolved issues from the past and provides the opportunity to identify and separate their own personal issues from those of their clients. Personal therapy also provides opportunities for the trainee to reflect upon and explore their unconscious process, for example that of countertransference (Freud, 1910); the emotional responses that arise from past experiences and that can become manifest within the therapeutic relationship.

I was fortunate that I was already in a consolidated therapeutic relationship with my therapist for many years prior to starting the training. Indeed, my experience of personal therapy strongly influenced my decision to begin my play therapy training. Over the years I have reflected much upon my different experiences of therapy in the past, where at times I have felt interrogated and questioned and at other times like some kind of case study. This reflection has helped inform me as to the kind of therapist that I would like to become.

Trainees are taken to a place of reflection that perhaps they do not think they need, or to places they simply do not want to revisit, but experiential activities and personal therapy provide the context within which these experiences can be explored and understood. Experiential process, set within a clear theoretical framework, is facilitated by a teaching approach that shows openness and acceptance to all that the trainees bring to the training experience. It is this process that facilitates the empowerment of the trainees to feel safe enough to use self-reflection and become aware of their feelings, by making links between aspects of the training and their own experiences and exploring their own vulnerabilities. Ultimately, this can lead the trainee to a place of acceptance.

In the second year of the training, we participate in an art psychotherapy workshop and we were given an instruction to create a visual image of the masculine side of our identity. I started drawing circles in the paper and ended up with nine circles joined by waves of different colours. It was an abstract image that I enjoyed drawing, losing myself in the process and just freely flowing with the chalk. When asked to reflect upon the work, I said that it reminded me of my father because the waves represented the flowing of music, something that he really enjoyed. To my surprise, one of my peers commented that my image looked like a uterus. I took my work home and looked at it later. It was clear what I expressed unconsciously and I felt "pushed" to face something that I did not want to. It was the unconscious emotional reality of my uterus being my masculine side as it felt to me, in the moment, as being unable to nurture and contain.

This kind of experimental activity, alongside personal therapy, helped me to explore in some depth the emotional implications of my miscarriage. It was very important for me to identify the unconscious idea of not being able to "hold" or "contain" and how this was expressed through my need to "control" external situations. In relation to my practice, I started my practice placement wanting to know everything and do everything right, as if it were a mechanism to cope with the painful uncertainty of loss.

Although I recognise myself as a very reflective individual, it was difficult for me to truly connect with that aspect of my experience and it was taking me to a place where I did not feel genuine, because my response at times of emotional struggle has always been to work. As painful as it was to recognise that, and allow myself to cry and be angry, and ask a 100 times "why", it was a liberating experience that allowed me to give to myself. Once I was able to observe and embrace these feelings, I was able to relate to my clients in a more relaxed and genuine manner and was able to understand my own process in relation to their experiences.

As a trainee, there was a gradual rather than a sudden shift in the development of my self-awareness and acceptance during the programme, helped by a sense of normalisation gained from the group experience, a process I was much more aware of during the second year of my training. The experience of witnessing another's vulnerability enabled me to relate to my own vulnerability in a safe way, within a shared and non-judgemental context. For trainees, this is important as it allows them to reflect and understand their emotional defences and embrace their feelings of vulnerability, rather than hide or push them away. In turn, this can help trainees develop the core skills of congruence, genuineness and authenticity. The sense of *not being the only one who struggles*, alongside the mutual support felt within the group, validates their own experience, proving the emotional context in which they develop self-acceptance and consequently feel more accepting of others. This can be a turning point within the training and highlights the development of self-awareness and the core conditions as conceptualised by Rogers (2003) of congruence, acceptance and unconditional positive regard.

## Final words

Many years ago, I became aware of the art of Kintsugi (Santini, 2019), also known as Kintsukuroi, which means "mending with gold". It is a technique developed in Japan during the 15th century and involves repairing a broken object by stressing its cracks in gold. This practice holds the symbolism of resilience and healing, a symbolism that encourages us to exceed our battles and transform our sufferings into something precious.

Reflecting on this process and the symbolism of the Kintsugi art makes me conclude that this experience is something that will always inform my professional practice as vulnerability is not something about which we should feel ashamed of. Hiding or negating vulnerabilities will only aid to weaken the meaning of our own struggles, and in the professional field, will undermine the aptitude to validate and respect the struggle of the clients.

The journey of the training did not prevent me from encountering strong feelings. I fell apart but was able to put back together the pieces of "my story", identifying with my sense of truth, a truth that feels like identity. I realised that with the ability to be still and allow myself to feel, I was able to activate the wisdom within me. This is when "the process" took form in my experience and the phrase "trust the process" crystallised.

## References

Aguilera, M. (2009) *An Exploratory Study of the Developmental Experience of Novice Play Therapists*. http://hdl.handle.net/1957/11534.

Axline, V. (2002) *Play Therapy*. Edinburgh: Elsevier Health Sciences.

Blanco, P., et al. (2014) Understanding the Concept of Genuineness in Play Therapy: Implications for the Supervision and Teaching of Beginning Play Therapists. *International Journal of Play Therapy*, 24(1), pp. 44–54.

Brown, B. (2015) *Daring Greatly. How the Courage to Be Vulnerable Transforms the Way We Live, Love, Parent and Lead*. New York: Penguin Random House.

Freud, S. (1910) *The Future Prospects of Psycho-Analytic Therapy*. The Standard Edition of the Complete Psychological Works of Sigmund Freud (vol. XI, pp. 139–151). London: Hogarth Press.

Landreth, G. (2012) *Play Therapy: The Art of the Relationship* (3rd ed.). New York: Brunner-Routledge.

Le Vay, D. & Cuschieri, E. (2016) *Challenges in the Theory and Practice of Play Therapy*. London. Routledge.

Luft, J. & Ingham, H. (1955) The Johari Window, a Graphic Model of Interpersonal Awareness. In: *Proceedings of the Western Training Laboratory in Group Development*. Los Angeles: UCLA.

Moustakas, C. (1990) *Heuristic Research: Design, Methodology and Applications*. London. Sage Publications.

Moustakas, C. (2007) *Relationship Play Therapy*. Lanham: Rowman & Littlefield Publishers.

Oxford Living Dictionary (2017) Available at: https://www.lexico.com/definition/vulnerability (accessed July 2020).

Rogers, C. (2003) *Client-Centered Therapy*. London: Constable & Robinson Ltd.

Rønnestad, M. & Skovholt, T. (2003) The Journey of the Counsellor and Therapist: Research Findings and Perspectives on Professional Development. *Journal of Career Development*, 30(1), pp. 5–44.

Santini, C. (2019) *Kintsugi: Finding Strength in Imperfection*. Kansas City: Andrews McMeel Publishing.

Chapter 9

# Self-care

## Another important relationship

*Sue Topping*

Rest and self-care are so important. When you take time to replenish your spirit, it allows you to serve others from the overflow. You cannot serve from an empty vessel.

(Eleanor Brownn, 2013)

### Self-care: what is it all about?

It is something we hear about regularly. It is something we know we need to do. It is something that we refer to in clinical supervision. But what actually is self-care? How do we do it properly? My experience of self-care has been, and continues to be, a journey of exploration and curiosity rather than one of mastery. Having studied this as a topic during my master's thesis, I perhaps know a little more than most. However, this knowledge and understanding does not always translate into the ability to practice self-care successfully.

When I undertook a course of study to become a child-centred play therapist, I had not fully appreciated the attention that should be paid to oneself, in order to remain psychologically healthy. Self-care had been mentioned during my training, in personal therapy and during clinical supervision, yet the more I explored and experimented with it, the more inadequate my attempts felt. Most therapists would argue that there is a critical need to participate actively in self-care. However, the practical challenges and barriers that many play therapists face while trying to carve out time and space for self-replenishment are very real. It is essential to be aware of the implications of compassion fatigue, secondary trauma and burnout as well as the strong ethical requirement of our professional body to engage in self-care.

But do play therapists need greater coaching, training and mentoring in the art of self-care, given its importance and the need to develop it as a skill? – A question we probably all know the answer to. My motivation at this point in my career is to understand where the vulnerabilities of therapists lie and identify the challenges of maintaining psychological health within a therapist role, in order to maintain professional competence and ethically sound practice.

I have also reflected upon the intrinsic link between self-care and self-worth and have attempted to understand the theoretical psychophysiological evidence

DOI: 10.4324/9781003017271-9

available that can help us to understand the challenges faced by therapists. I certainly recognise the barriers I have encountered personally, and this exploration has enabled me to understand why I find it difficult to be kinder to myself and to give myself permission to self-care. Acknowledging this aspect of my journey has enabled me to begin to participate more effectively in self-care experiences, and whilst I still have work to do, my learning has provided a scaffold upon which to develop my practice as a play therapist.

Drawing upon some of my heuristic research (Moustakas, 1990) and personal experience of self-care in practice since qualifying, I will share my lived experiences of the relationship I now have with self-care and the ongoing battle that remains between the moral dilemma of balancing my needs alongside the practical implications of time and the needs of others. My hopes for this chapter are to share my experience with play therapy professionals who like me, on occasion, struggle with the practicalities of applying self-care. I do not have all the answers, but perhaps by sharing my experience and unanswered questions, we can begin a dialogue within the play therapy community.

## My self-care journey

I became motivated by this topic when, during my play therapy training, I unexpectedly became seriously ill, overnight, with no warning. One day I went to bed thinking about the topic of my next essay and the next day I was rushed to a specialist London hospital with a Subarachnoid Haemorrhage (a brain aneurysm). My life was turned upside down within the blink of an eye and I was forced to take a long sabbatical to recover (much to my displeasure at the time). Whilst I am now well, I have had to address my unhealthy work/life balance and embrace new ways of managing my day-to-day life. Migraines and fatigue are now a feature of daily living that can impact on my effectiveness to practice as a play therapist, so I have had to develop ways to maintain my professional and ethical responsibilities. As I navigate the balance between being a "good enough" play therapist and my internal needs, I now try to embrace self-care more effectively and consider more openly what it really means to put myself first.

My journey through self-care has certainly been a bumpy and at times confusing one, beginning with a genuine desire to understand the motivation (or lack of) that has influenced my self-care practice and perhaps identify potential personal challenges and barriers. This is where my heuristic research study (Moustakas,1990) into this question has been of considerable benefit to my comprehension and understanding of self-care. The term "heuristic" was coined by Moustakas (1990: 9) from the Greek expression *heuriskein* (to "discover" or "find"). The philosophy behind this was to develop a research methodology that could capture lived human experience. Moustakas makes clear that the essential principles of the approach are based on autobiographical discovery of a phenomenon examined by the researcher. Through this in-depth exploration of lived experience, the researcher gains greater understanding, knowledge and consciousness of the topic being investigated.

Heuristic research is recognised as a scientific approach designed to sensitively capture the thoughtful gatherings of idiosyncratic experience and behaviour of subjects. A researcher's continued inquisitiveness towards their own experience and that of their co-researchers fuels the search for further understanding of the subjective. For the purpose of this chapter and to maintain anonymity, I will not be including findings from co-researchers involved in my study.

Moustakas (1990: 39) identifies three main qualities essential to heuristic investigation; "concentrated gazing" in a bid to pursue meaning, "focus on a topic" to provide clear, precise and tangible focus of inquiry, and "methods" that scaffold the gathering, scrutiny and fusion of data. Heuristic research requires methods that are creative and expressive rather than the more traditional approaches to quantitative data gathering, as they are more suited to capturing and searching for meaning within experience. I therefore used personal reflections via journals and discussion, as well as imagery and symbolism. My journaling was supported by informal discussions with peers, family, my personal therapist and mentor throughout the study. The creative mediums enabled me to explore particular behaviours that were more challenging to embrace cognitively, and so through the use of sand trays, art materials, quotes, music and poems, I was able to facilitate a deep process of personal exploration, supported by these heuristic research approaches that began to unlock deep feelings and emotions related to self-care.

Self-care is so important to a wide range of caring professions (Skovholt & Trotter-Mathison, 2016) yet it could be suggested that self-care can be a rather elusive concept, which if ignored can affect the well-being and professional competence of any practicing therapist. Due to the scarcity of research within child-centred play therapy specifically, I also explored the allied professions of counselling and psychotherapy, and the umbrella term "helping professions" to fully understand self-care.

## Terminology and definitions of self-care

When reviewing definitions of self-care, the overriding theme that appeared is one of "taking action" in the care of self (Oxford University Press, 2017). This appears to take the form of varying activities or pastimes, but the need to take personal responsibility remains central. Within the caring professions, it is acknowledged that therapists do not always lead by example and attention is drawn to the professional and ethical priorities that underpin a therapist's capacity to practice in the care of others (Parsons & Zhang, 2014). The British Association of Play Therapists (2020), ethical principle C, "Non-Maleficence", clearly states that therapists should "not provide services when unfit to do so due to personal impairment, including illness, personal circumstances or intoxication". Whilst in training, I found this responsibility overwhelming at times with copious self-care strategies on offer, and little time to fully embrace any of them. As Parsons and Zhang (2014: 285) point out, "self-care should not, and cannot, begin once you start your professional life".

There is a considerable amount of literature that explores strategies for self-care, covering key areas of the physical, psychological, emotional, spiritual and the professional self (Parsons & Zhang, 2014). The overwhelming message is one of creating balance between caring for others and the self. Identifying what self-care is and possible ways to achieve it is only a small part of the conundrum, understanding why it is needed and what prevents engagement with it is another.

The starting point in my research process was a basic mind map asking a series of questions that, at the time, filled my sphere of cognitive processing (Fig. 9.1).

These questions formed a starting point as I began to explore literature and have informal conversations with peers. My first journal entry (Fig. 9.2) quickly identified the difficulty of finding balance, as well as an intrinsic inability to put myself before others, referring to being "incapable of embracing it [self-care] successfully over a sustained period of time". My thoughts had completely been overtaken by self-care and I recall finding the topic emerging in almost all areas of my life. I reflected in my journal that finding the words to articulate my thoughts had been extremely challenging. I turned to the other mediums outlined, recognising the need to capture less cognitive and more emotionally felt experiences.

As my exploration progressed and life pressures mounted, I became increasingly frustrated by my attempts to practice self-care and always found myself falling short. I recognised the need and value of self-care, but barriers kept getting in the way. I chose to create a piece of artwork called "Frustration" to try and express my displeasure at the situation I found myself in, as I knew that I had a battle on my hands and needed an emotional outlet (Fig. 9.3.).

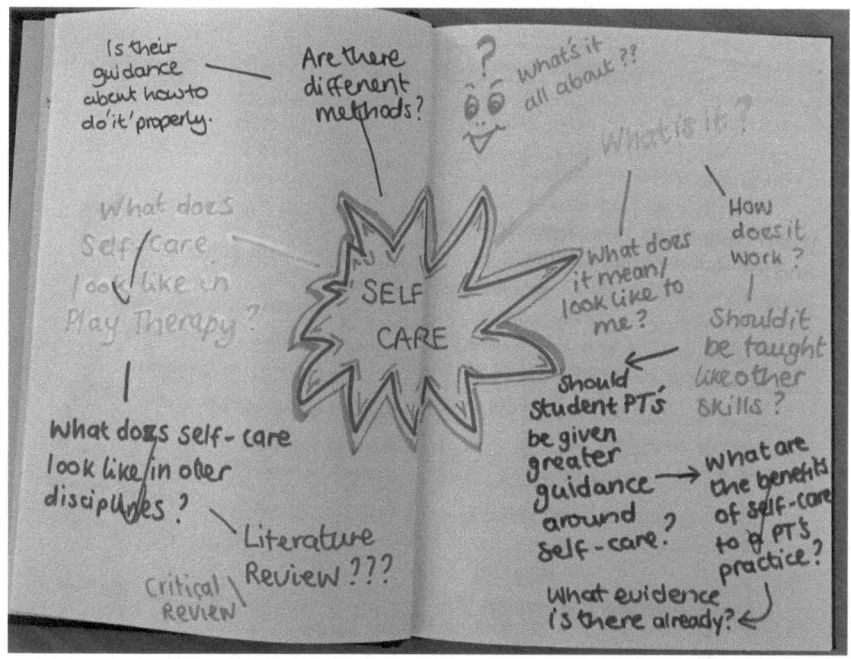

*Figure 9.1* Mind map

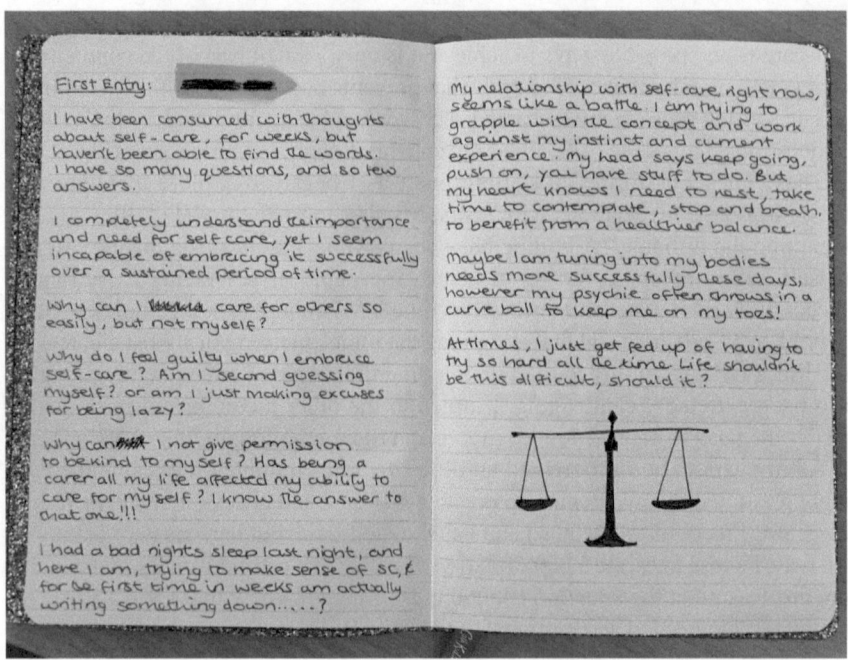

*Figure 9.2* Journal Entry One

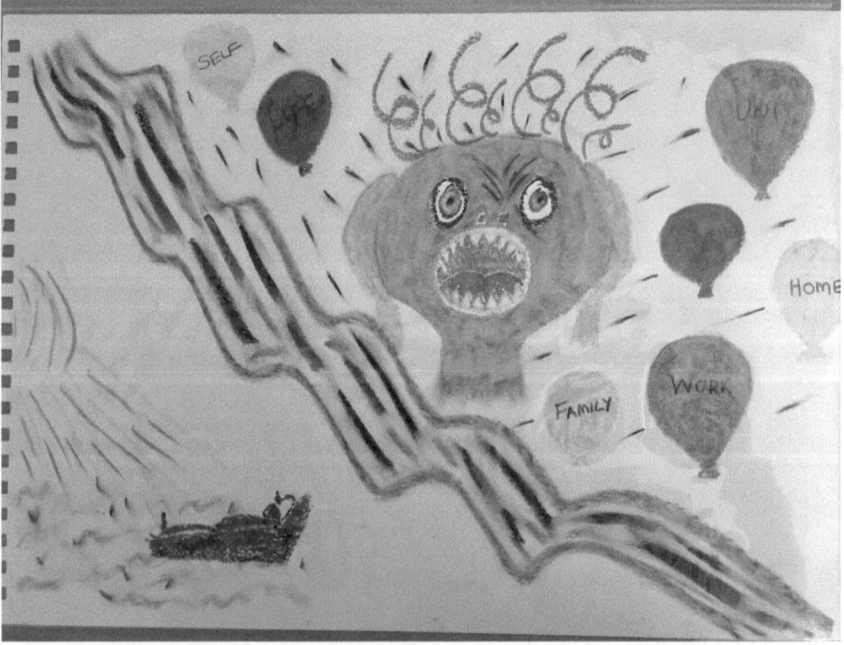

*Figure 9.3* Frustration

My intention with this image was to capture life's reality in the top half along-side all the challenges that float around, with the desire for self-care in the lower half and a vast space in between that is often impassable, reflecting the unobtain-able target of self-care. Similar feelings of frustration were also captured in a journal entry (Fig. 9.4.) in which I expressed annoyance at the challenges and expectations of others, interfering with what I felt I needed. I began questioning my ability to express my needs to others as well as the realisation that self-care is

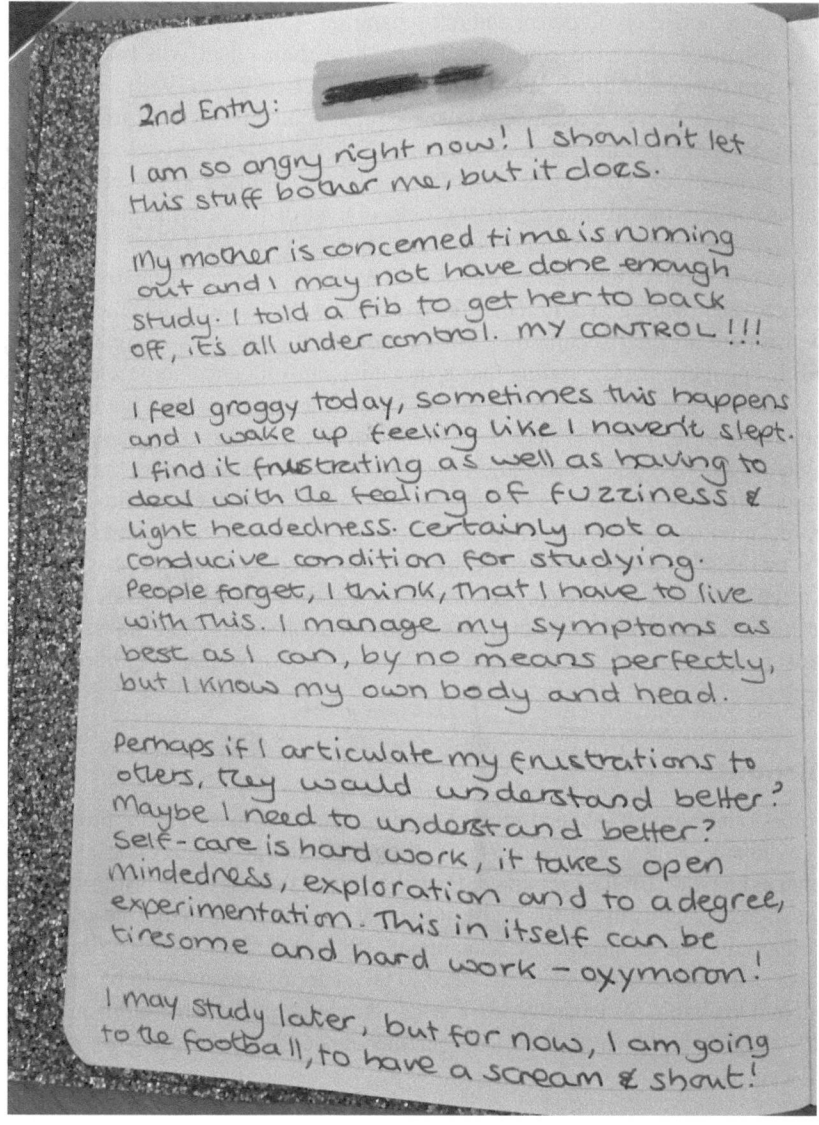

*Figure 9.4* Journal Entry Two

hard work, requiring open mindedness, exploration and, to a degree, experimentation. This felt tiresome and something of an oxymoron.

## The caring cycle

Whilst grappling with my own demons and barriers to self-care, I began exploring some of the difficulties associated with poor self-care practice. The concept of the "Caring Cycle" originates from Skovholt (2005), who linked together seven sources of data from the counselling process, attachment theory and practitioner application. Skovholt developed a cyclical model around three elements, "empathic attachment, active involvement and felt separation" (Skovholt, 2005: 86).

A therapist's ability to empathically attach to their client will be dependent upon their own attachment experiences as an infant. Bowlby's (1988) work identifies the importance of experiencing successful attachments, as they are crucial to human relationships and later adult functioning. As Bowlby suggests, "to make intimate emotional bonds with other individuals, sometimes in the care seeking role and sometimes in the caregiving one, is regarded as a principal feature of effective personality functioning and mental health" (1988: 136).

Skovholt (2005: 86) points out that for therapists who have experienced repeated challenging attachments, the process of "empathic attachment, active involvement and felt separation" will be problematic, potentially causing stress and disengagement. He claims that a therapist can influence some elements of the caring dimension, namely the quality of their engagement and having expert knowledge of the client's issues, for example difficulties with anxiety, self-esteem or confidence. As the therapeutic relationship develops and the therapist feels competent, they experience a sensation of increased satisfaction with a greater appreciation of their achievement. Skovholt (2005: 87) proposes that the success of a therapist's intervention can be wholly influenced by the three phases of the "Caring Cycle". It could be argued that the engagement and knowledge elements outlined by Skovholt (2005) may seem somewhat challenging at times, and that pressures placed upon the "Caring Cycle" could lead to symptoms of burnout and compassion fatigue.

## Burnout

Professional burnout is a common phenomenon within many caring professions (Skovholt & Trotter-Mathison, 2016), triggering anxiety, depression and emotional exhaustion for the individual. It can be argued that the cause originates from two sources of mismatch for the professional, a "loss of meaning in caring for another and loss of therapeutic attachment" (Skovholt, 2005: 83). To limit these losses, we must first recognise the need to take care of ourselves, to be fully present and available for those we work with. Skovholt and Trotter-Mathison (2016: 127) suggest that "we need to lose our innocence about the need for assertive self-care".

Freudenberger (1975) formed the term burnout in a professional context, when he identified three key features; becoming emotionally overwhelmed, a reducing sense of achievement and an inability to connect fully with the attributes of a therapeutic relationship. The therapeutic attributes described by Rogers (1951, 1980) of unconditional positive regard, empathy and congruence become increasingly challenging to uphold when being placed under pressure by the features of burnout. This can lead to the therapist questioning themselves, their approaches and even their professional calling. Skovholt and Trotter-Mathison (2016: 103) refer to a "profound weariness and haemorrhaging of the self" that is recognised by the psychotherapy community and allied caring professions.

It is also useful to acknowledge that there are two forms of burnout identified by Skovholt; "meaning burnout" and "caring burnout" (2016: 108). The first, put simply, refers to the loss of motivation in working with the chosen client group in a caring role. The second relates to connectedness with clients, a process of "professional attachment – involvement – separation – re-creation" (2016: 108). Both forms contribute to the overwhelming feeling of disconnection from the work, which can lead to ineffective practice.

During the Coronavirus pandemic, the response in the United Kingdom to COVID-19 was to lock down the country between December 2020 and March 2021. During this time, my practice moved completely onto an online platform, which presented a whole range of challenges and new experiences that I had not previously considered, for example screen fatigue and the reliability of an Internet connection. I felt a real sense of burnout for the first time in my career, and although I had read about it and understood it, I struggled to prevent it from happening to me. I felt the overwhelming need to contribute something, to support vulnerable children and their families through a terrifying ordeal, whilst still recognising and maintaining professional and ethical boundaries.

Once work began online, I quickly became awash with feelings of isolation, powerful transference and of being too distant from the client (metaphorically and physically). I regularly questioned my practice; if it was enough, if it was right for each child, and I utilised clinical supervision and personal therapy throughout. At no point however did I consider if the work I was doing was right for me. I did recognise that the online format was not ideal, but it was better than nothing, both for my own sanity and for the children I was working with.

Other than these surface reflections, I was unable at the time to reflect any deeper whilst in the "eye of the storm" and believe I was in a state of faux functioning, if you will, an additional human survival response that kicked in within me to find a way of coping during this unprecedented time. In this state, I felt that I was functioning sufficiently in the face of adversity whilst containing the children with whom I was working. The children came to no harm and in all cases felt held during this period and were able to re-enter their personal processes almost seamlessly. However, when I reflected afterwards on that period of time, I realised that I had experienced burnout – questioning my ability, what I was doing, how I was doing it and, on some occasions, why I was doing it. I was unable to undertake effective restorative practice such as adequate sleep, exercise, diet, balanced relationships, hobbies, community and spirituality (Davis Bush, 2015). Put simply, outside of the sessions I was exhausted; my vessel was empty and the simplest of tasks became increasingly challenging.

Baker (2003: 13) suggests that the key components of self-care are "self-awareness, self-regulation and balance" yet I was clearly unable to comprehend this at the time. I had not learnt or been taught what to do in this situation and neither had any therapist, teacher or nurse across the world. So, what drove me to continue? What was so powerful that it blatantly and unapologetically circumvented my own needs, with the needs of others? I believe that it could have been one of the less cognitive aspects of psychophysiology highlighted by Rothschild and Rand (2006: 3) that activated three neuropsychological areas that they refer to as "mechanisms operating in interpersonal empathy", "autonomic nervous system arousal regulation" and "balanced functioning of brain structures providing clear thinking". In other words, my body needed me to continue to function in a therapeutic way in order that I could experience some level of functioning, by connecting with others through interpersonal empathy. I believe that my autonomic nervous system was able to regulate itself, to a degree, through the faux functioning belief that I was working and doing my bit, providing me with purpose. This in turn gave the illusion of clear thinking from time to time, that provided much-needed meaning to the strange experience we were all living through. What I should have done in relation to psychological self-care was powerfully overtaken by my psychophysiological needs.

In their comprehensive study of neurobiology and psychology, Rothschild and Rand (2006) signpost scientific evidence to support the theory that the therapist's risk of poor well-being can be reduced significantly by understanding the response of the brain and body, for example the neurobiology of empathy suggests that mirror neurons fire in the brain of one individual "reflect[ing] the activity of another's brain cells" (Rothschild & Rand, 2006: 42).

Throughout their book, Rothschild and Rands provide a range of exercises for therapists to explore and begin to understand their own psychophysiology so that interventions and skill-building can be tailored to suit individual need. This provides a less cognitive and more practical emphasis on the need to pay attention to how our body responds to others within the therapeutic relationship.

The complexity of managing self-care is influenced by a wide variety of factors, which take time to identify, explore and master, so perhaps it should be acknowledged that during a worldwide pandemic, when the fear of the unknown is at its greatest, self-care was possibly a step too far whilst immersed in the experience. Reflection and knowledge after the fact are sometimes all we have available to us so that we can make sense of the darkest of times. Remember, I said this was not easy!

## Compassion fatigue

Compassion fatigue is often considered alongside burnout. However, it is particularly distinctive due to the therapists' repeated exposure to traumatic suffering and anguish shared by clients (Skovholt & Trotter-Mathison, 2016). Figley (1995) identifies four reasons why those engaged in therapeutic roles are more prone to compassion fatigue: empathy, personal trauma, unresolved trauma and child trauma. The process of empathising with another's trauma makes the therapist susceptible to the trauma shared. A therapist's personal experience of trauma may be similar to that experienced by a client, and potential unresolved trauma from previous experience could trigger unhelpful emotions. Due to the confrontational and emotive nature of child trauma itself, there is a significant imbalance created for the therapist, impacting on their ability to refresh between clients and on their capacity to enter the Cycle of Caring outlined previously.

Large-scale research conducted by Woodward-Myers and Cornille (2002: 44) with professionals working with traumatised children identified that those with prolonged exposure and experience with this client group (more than one year) reported higher rates of "obsessive compulsive symptoms", "nervous tensions, panic attacks and feelings of terror". It was also noted that female workers experienced elevated "anger, irritability, jumpiness, exaggerated startle response, trouble concentrating, hypervigilance, nightmares, intrusive thoughts and images" (2002: 49).

To date, I have been fortunate not to experience any of the difficulties outlined in relation to compassion fatigue, possibly due to the detailed work I have completed in personal therapy to address my own childhood trauma. I am able to differentiate between my own experience and those shared metaphorically or symbolically in the playroom and have developed an additional level of understanding through undertaking eye movement desensitisation and reprocessing (EMDR) therapy (Shapiro, 2007) that has enabled me to connect with and process negative emotions and reframe them into positive ones. This has afforded me the opportunity to explore complex trauma in a more felt sense and therefore at a deeper level. For me, personal therapy has been a critical part of my self-care practice and whilst this could be considered as an expensive tool, the financial outlay is by far outweighed by the deeper insight I have gained, so I will remain an advocate of this approach.

## Challenges and pitfalls of self-care practice

The balance between care of the self and care for others requires continual monitoring, to identify therapist vulnerability to life pressures and stress. Selye (1974: 62) describes an "altruistic egotism" that forms the basis of nature, a code for all living beings to survive within eco-systems. He suggests that the purpose of this is to provide a code of conduct encompassing acceptable norms that are innate to our own and others' survival. Caring for ourselves is therefore as crucial to our own existence as it is to whom we are helping. Yet those in the helping professions often overlook their own needs, thus dampening the "altruistic egotism" need, giving rise to potential problems.

Rothschild and Rand (2006) identify that one of the key attributes of a therapist is the ability to empathise with their client. This is widely acknowledged as a crucial element of the therapeutic relationship and the foundation upon which all work with the individual will then flourish. As Rothschild and Rand (2006: 10) acknowledge, "empathy is our major, greatest, and most reliable tool". They also point out, however, that empathy could be regarded as our Achilles heel, that if unchecked could "threaten our well-being at times" (2006: 10). In their hypothesis of the relationship between empathy and possible damage to the therapist, Rothschild and Rand (2006: 11) identify the danger of "unconscious empathy", a way of being that the therapist is unaware of or able to regulate. They believe that this is at the root of, or at the very least, has an association with, compassion fatigue and burnout. This may go some way towards understanding the subjective nature of this topic, and the battle that takes place between the therapist and the practical application of self-care.

Whilst exploring this conundrum, I often found it challenging to find words, so I created some free form artwork, without too much cognitive thought, that captured my feelings at this time (Figs. 9.5 and 9.6). These depictions were initially formed as part of an unrelated activity during my training but became relevant to the battle I was having with myself and those around me.

Figure 9.5, called "Pressure", reflects the weight I sometimes felt when things, such as expectation, push down on me and squeeze out any space I may have carved out for self-care. The disappearing face in the centre captures the all-consuming power of the needs of others.

Figure 9.6, called "Smothered", is an expression of all the "other stuff" that comes before I can even begin to consider myself – the feeling of being smothered and unable to function in any coherent form. I later discovered that addressing these battles, particularly those with myself, provided some objectivity and clarity. However, before reaching this point, my hand was once again forced due to a virus which landed me in bed for several days. In Figure 9.7, I began exploring the relationship between taking on-board self-care and then experiencing some form of negative consequence afterwards, for example missing deadlines. I considered if this was anything to do with my attitude or frame of reference and pondered whether other play therapists experienced this. I acknowledged the need to resist the pressure to beat myself up and slowly catch up despite this sitting uncomfortably.

Baker (2003: 13) suggests that the key components of self-care are "self-awareness, self-regulation and balance". She explains that self-awareness can be challenging and hostile, as the therapist explores their inner struggles and pressures, exposing their needs in a crude form. An awareness of our own needs provides us with the opportunity to consider and process them adequately. Failure to do so is likely to lead to detrimental behaviours spilling over into our practice or even suppressed needs infecting our relationships with clients (Baker, 2003). It is however

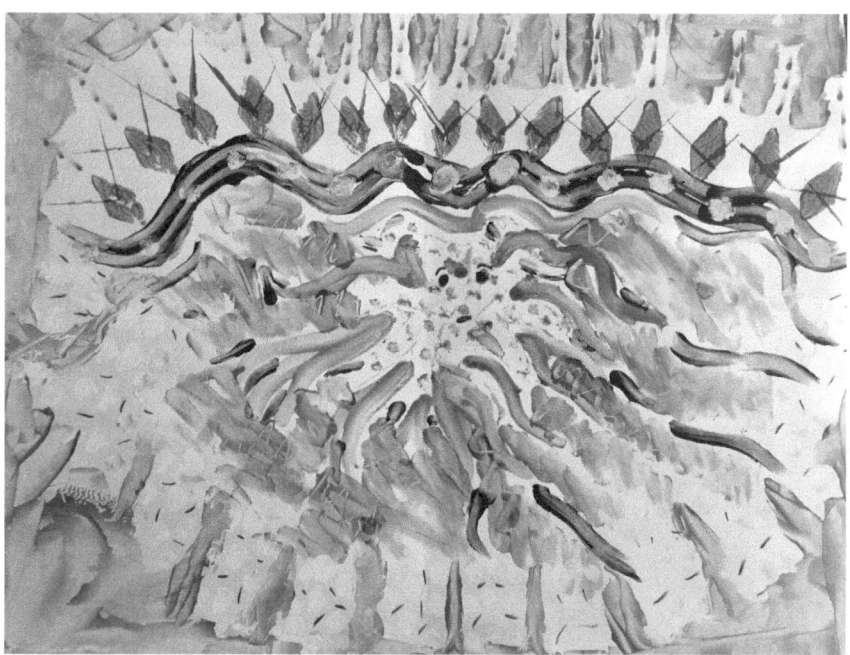

*Figure 9.5* Pressure

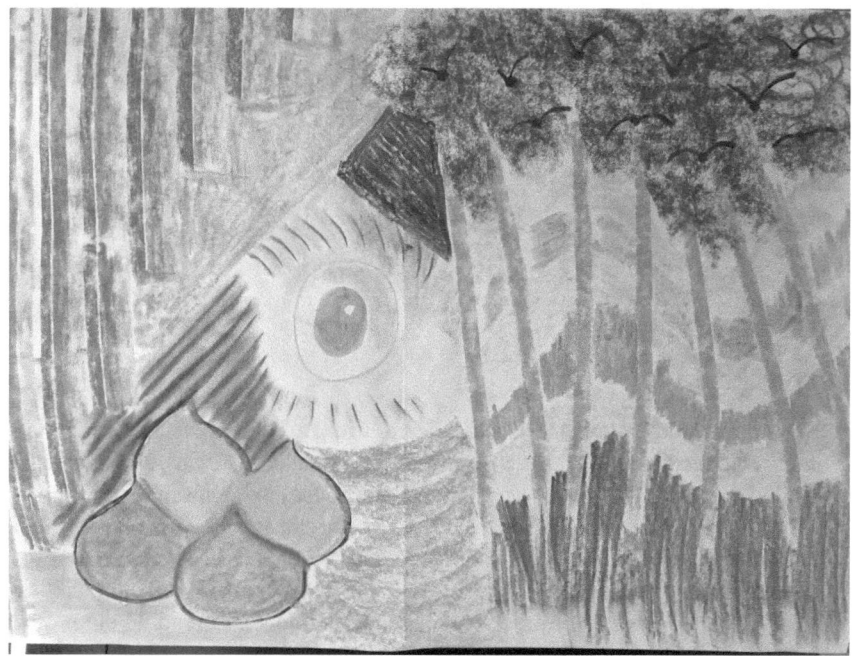

*Figure 9.6* Smothered

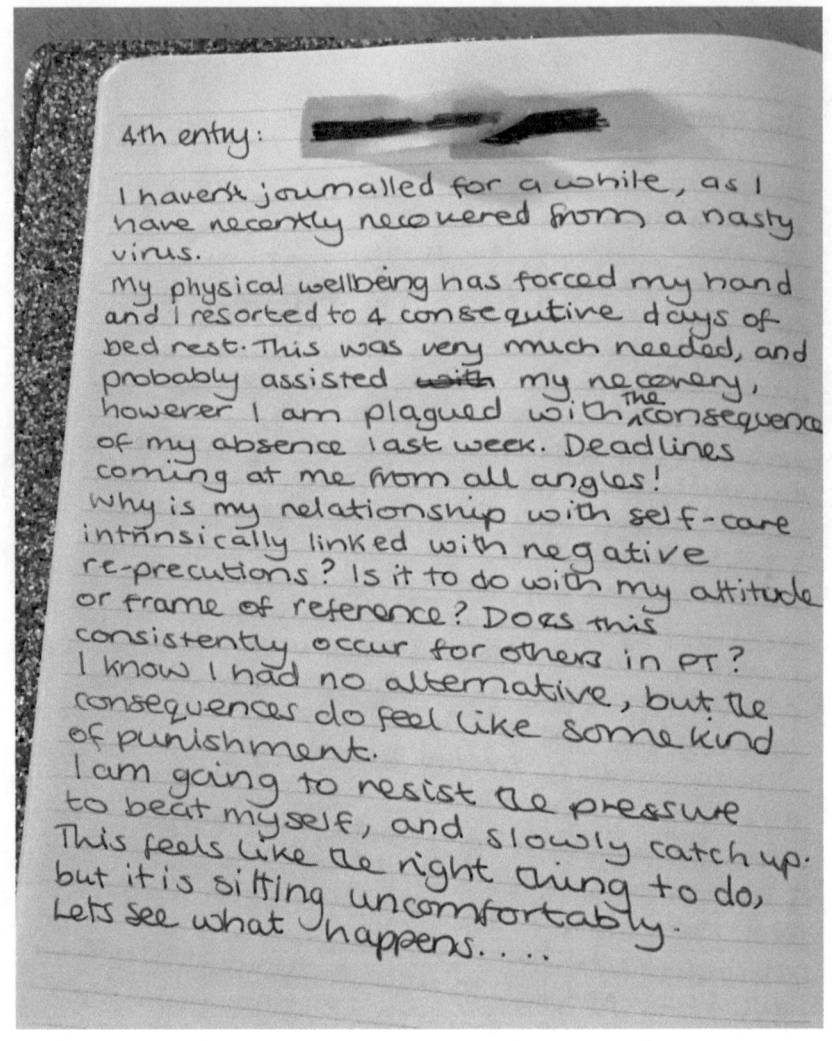

*Figure 9.7* Journal Entry Four

important that self-awareness is considered from a compassionate viewpoint, avoiding a judgemental or self-deprecating stance. Baker's (2003) views on self-regulation require the therapist to adapt their responses to cognisant and intuitive stimuli, considering alternative activities such as relaxation and fitness, to help find emotional inner balance. Our ability to self-regulate derives from our skills in managing impulsive reactions, a sense of self-worth and our personal welfare (Baker, 2003). The more we practice self-regulation under pervading emotional agitation, the more we become aware "of our feelings, needs and limits" (Baker, 2003: 15). The final element, balance, referred to by Baker as a battle between dualisms, represents the interface between conflicting influences within us, for example "action and rest; doing and being and work and play" (2003: 16). The term balance is regularly used, but is often a tricky skill to acquire, needing to be accomplished and sustained repeatedly. In the search to find the centre, a point of equilibrium, Baker explains that the process requires regular fluctuation and alteration. A feeling of accomplishment, mastery and esteem can be felt, enabling a capacity to care for self.

My relationship with self-care fluctuated between frustration and early acceptance during my studies and at times sometimes still does today. An opportunity to contemplate my self-care journey appeared in the form of a workshop, where I created a sand tray, later named "Contemplation" (Fig. 9.8). I felt that I was beginning to grapple with and accept the challenges of self-care, whilst at the same time beginning to experience the benefit of the activities I had achieved. Watching live football, meeting friends for a cup of tea or a meal, spending time with animals, personal therapy and clinical supervision all became more prominent features as useful self-care tools that I still utilise today.

Skovholt and Trotter-Mathison (2016) refer to the "Four Dimensions of Health" encompassing a balance between physical, emotional/social, intellectual

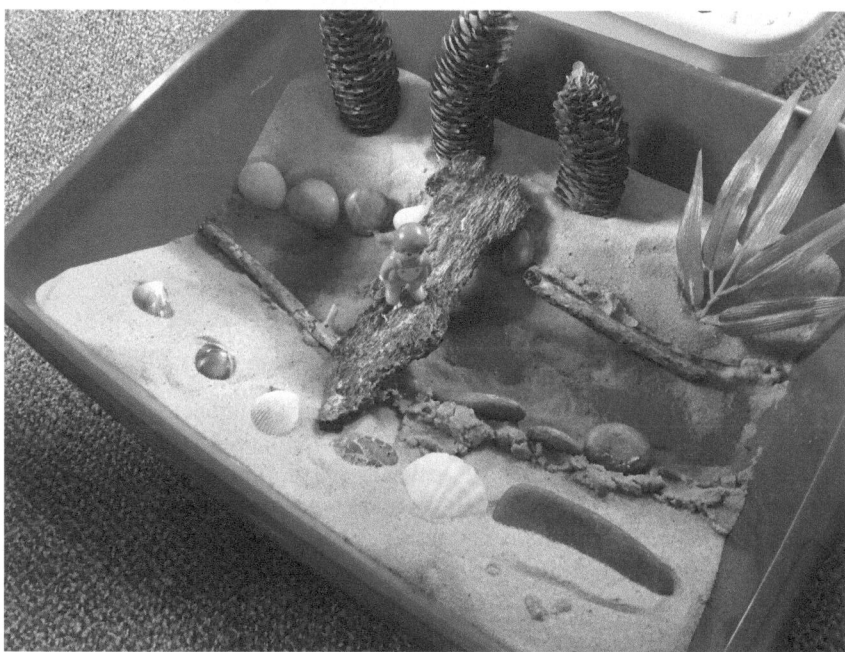

*Figure 9.8* Contemplation

and spiritual health. Portrayed diagrammatically as a diamond, they state that the "diamond symbolises the reality that the whole is greater than the sum of the parts. Yet, the whole is strong only by attending to each dimension" (2016: 182).

There are many strategies and suggestions available to therapists to support ongoing self-care; however, finding methods that are successful is as much about knowing oneself, as experimenting with those that are helpful. The Meany-Walen et al. (2018) qualitative study of play therapist perception of self-care and tools utilised identified four main themes: "individual activities, interpersonal relationships, professional practices, play and intent" (Meany-Walen et al., 2018: 182). This sample group was randomly selected from the Association of Play Therapy and represented 10% of their membership. The study demonstrated that self-care was of great importance to the participants; however, 91% described their training as not preparing them for "wellness and self-care" (Meany-Walen et al., 2018: 183), which suggests a potential learning skills gap as identified from my own experience.

A further reflection that should also be noted is an acknowledgement of the restrictions placed around wellness and self-care activities during COVID-19 lockdowns in the United Kingdom. Both myself and, I am sure, many other therapists experienced a ". . . profound weariness and haemorrhaging of the self . . .". Mathison (2016: 103) recognised as symptoms of professional burnout (Freudenberger, 1975) during this period. Whilst I was unable to at the time, I have now identified the brutal suffocation of my preferred self-care tools imposed upon me for the greater good, which no doubt contributed to the feelings I experienced. I have since actively been re-introducing those tools that I am able to, within current restrictions and I strongly advise others to do the same, as there is a very real fatigue amongst peers and colleagues who are perhaps only now beginning to feel the consequences of the pressures we have faced together during the COVID-19 pandemic. The restrictions, in some form, are likely to remain or be reintroduced, so tangible solutions need to be identified for any therapist working under this pressure.

## Professional competence of the play therapist

Within therapeutic work, there is a clear expectation that professionals will follow ethical practice and a professional code of conduct to protect themselves and their clients. It seems helpful at this point to explore the similarities/differences between the major professional bodies that underpin play therapy, counselling and psychotherapy practice in the United Kingdom. I have identified and reviewed relevant documentation from two play therapy bodies, and three counselling/psychotherapy bodies for comparison. All the documentation reviewed highlights the responsibility of the therapist to maintain good psychological mental health, citing that failing to do so should result in reduction or cessation of practice until full health has returned. Although the wording may alter, the premise of all regulatory bodies reviewed identifies the professional conduct expected of therapists in establishing their fitness to practice.

It could perhaps be argued that play therapy is a growing profession with a relatively new professional body, the British Association of Play Therapists (BAPT) established in 1992, in comparison to the British Association of Counselling and Psychotherapists (BACP) and the United Kingdom Council for Psychotherapy (UKCP, 2009) both founded in 1977. However, Play Therapy United Kingdom (PTUK), which formed in 2000, has one of the more specific requirements, stating the need for therapists to consider "self-respect" and explore "life enhancing activities and relationships outside of therapeutic work" (PTUK, 2013: 10). The most explicit guidance regarding self-care comes from BACP, who cite care for self as one of the core principles of self-respect. They also refer to "a healthy balance between our work and other aspects of life" (British Association of Counselling and Psychotherapists, 2018: 30). Those who are the most ambiguous in relation to self-care seem to be BAPT and BCP who refer to being unfit due to "impairment, including illness, personal circumstances or intoxication" (British Association of Play Therapists, 2020: 3) and "physical or psychological health seriously impaired" along with the possible "effects of personal stress" (British Psychoanalytic Council, 2011: 5–6). The British Association of Play Therapists (2020: 8) also identifies in their Code of Good Practice in Play Therapy, "4.10. Personal issues and circumstances" that individuals should be mindful of their personal circumstances and how this may impact on their competence to practice. It appears that the extent of the experience of relevant founding bodies may not be the influence behind ambiguity of self-care and ethical principles. It should be pointed out that although BACP have defined self-care as important, none of the professional bodies specify self-care practice; instead, they only allude to it in a more general sense.

The presence of self-care advice and guidance available in the publication "Therapy Today: The Voice of the Counselling and Psychotherapy Profession" (Centre for Personal and Professional Development, 2017: 44) features a regular self-care topic written by a practising psychotherapist. Research into other professional journals found limited guidance. When speaking informally to therapists from other disciplines about their training, it seems that self-care is mentioned within their professional qualification, perhaps not in the detail that it deserves, but is identified as a critical area of practice. There is, however, a clear ethical need for therapists to be aware of self-care practice, to maintain their clinical competence, which is also an implied need within the BAPT code of ethics. It could be argued that self-care is a skill that can be taught as much as other therapeutic skills, so should it therefore be incorporated into the accredited training programmes currently available in the United Kingdom as a core component of training? Whilst I may not be able to answer this question, it does raise the issue as a subject for future consideration within the play therapy field.

## Reflections of self-care within the play therapy community

Having reviewed the information available about self-care in counselling, psychotherapy and the helping professions, I became curious about the dearth of literature and formal documented self-care practice within the play therapy profession specifically. This led me to wondering why it is not considered with greater importance within the field.

After a thorough search, I was able to find references, either directly or indirectly, to self-care. Ray (2011: 71) refers to the need for personal therapy throughout play therapy training and "over a lifetime of professional practice". She discusses the important elements of a therapeutic relationship between the child and the play therapist, acknowledging that experiencing unconditional positive regard, self-awareness and self-acceptance first-hand as part of one's own therapy is critical. Ray refers to the work of Wilkins (2016: 164), who identifies that if therapists do not pay attention to self-care, they will experience a "decreasing ability to be congruent" as a direct result of stress and burnout. Cochran et al. devote a chapter to the ongoing development of a child-centred play therapist, identifying that as individual practice develops, it is likely that the "core conditions of empathy, genuineness and unconditional positive regard" will be challenged, leading to signs of burnout (2010: 384). They cite the need for conscious and proactive attention to personal development, which can be achieved through a variety of methods including supervision, personal therapy, meditation, spirituality, being outdoors and socialising with family, friends or animals.

Landreth (2012: 103–104) discusses the need for "therapist self-understanding", where he promotes play therapist's responsibility to engage in intimate exploration of themselves and their motives through personal therapy, group therapy and supervision. He also acknowledges the need for self-acceptance for the therapist to remain fully accepting of the child.

Maschi (2015) specifically explores the risks and benefits for professionals working with children who have experienced trauma or crisis and advocates that satisfaction from this work is experienced more readily if practitioners actively engage in self-care. She eloquently highlights the helpful and healthy responses to empathy with a client and points out when the balance shifts to a place where negative impact is experienced. Using the headings of "general psychological distress; grief, mourning and chronic bereavement; countertransference; burnout; secondary trauma stress and compassion fatigue; and vicarious trauma" (2015: 398–402), she gives examples of the associated risks, describes methods to assess impact and considers strategies to limit its effect.

As my understanding of the research broadened, I began to see opportunities to question the topic further. Whilst attending a training workshop about self-care with my peers, I felt the time was right to test some of my musings. I had been contemplating some ideas for a while that had featured in personal therapy and although I cannot pinpoint the exact moment prior to the workshop, I had stumbled across a strong link between self-worth and self-care. It almost seemed too obvious to be significant, but as I found myself sharing this during the workshop, a small seed began to germinate.

Soon, something seemed to click into place. The more I thought about self-worth, the more sense I made of the difficulties I had been experiencing. At a similar time, I had worked through some significant issues in my personal therapy, and one became a catalyst for the other. I became able to challenge my motivation to put myself first and slowly began experiencing guilt-free self-care by doing simple things, including spending quiet time on my own, getting better quality sleep, reducing my workload, saying no to loved ones – all things I had previously struggled with.

I became able to reflect on my journey and consider my relationship with self-worth as captured in the small world and sand tray images (Figs. 9.9 and 9.10). Figure 9.9, "Journey", was initially a reflection of my training experience. However, I soon realised the similarities the images held with my exploration of self-care. The early stages were challenging, twisting and turning, and occasionally messy (represented by the snake, vehicles and pink object). I then felt that self-care was all encompassing and sometimes wanted to hide away (shown in the image as a shell and yellow object). I then became able to explore the battle I was having with the uncomfortable parts of my relationship with self-care (represented by the animals and the red and green figures). The final part of my

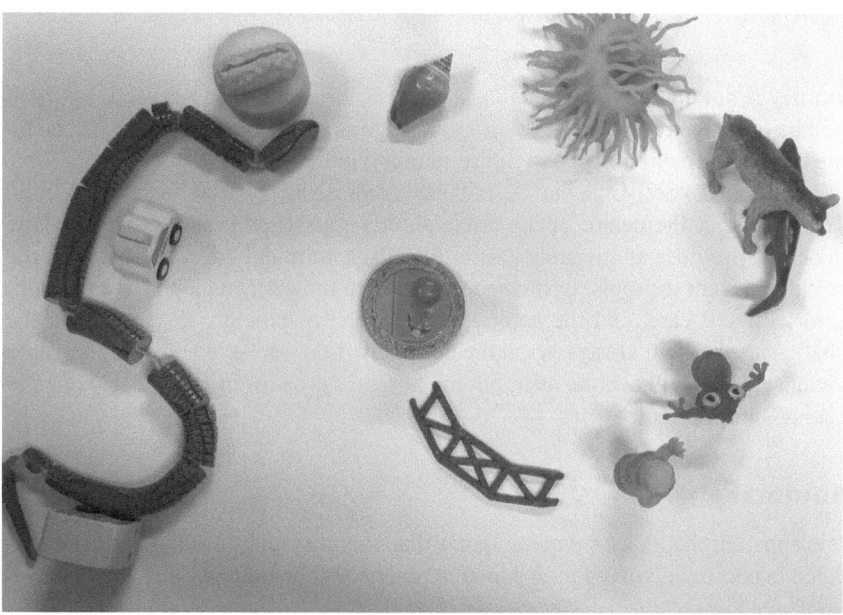

*Figure 9.9* Journey

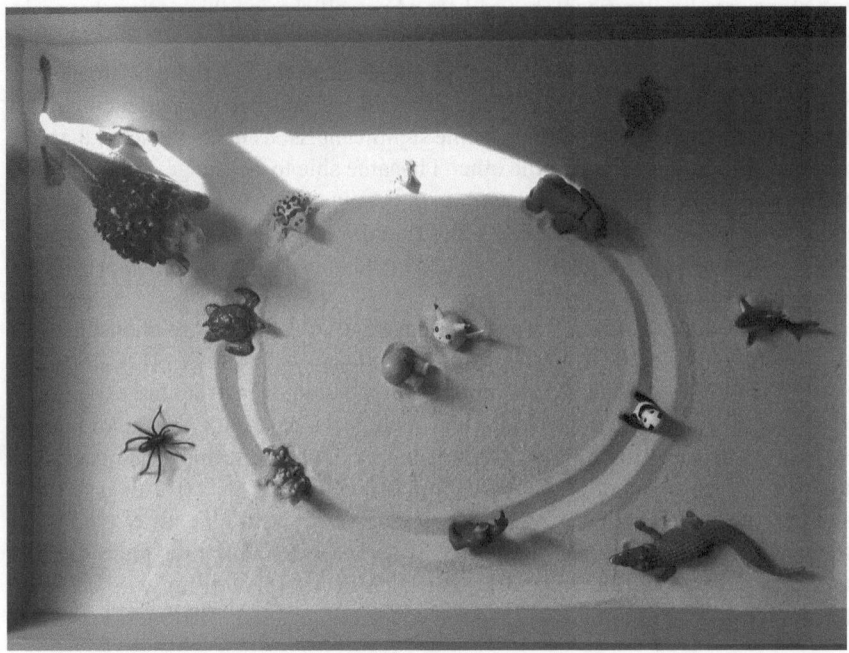

*Figure 9.10* Self-care and self-worth

journey is not complete, but there is a clearer path towards self-reflection, which will be of huge benefit as I develop and change as a play therapist (represented by the brown footpath, mirror and figure standing in the centre).

Figure 9.10, "Self-Care and Self-Worth", represents my relationship with both. The figures in the centre of the circle signify myself and my self-worth while the circle provides an invisible barrier of self-care around me. The figures on the circle represent the tools, or the people that help me maintain a positive relationship with self-care, and the animals circling the outside are a reminder of the challenges that will always be on the periphery. I do not believe that my learning about self-care will ever be over, but my horizons are now broadened and open to change or opportunity.

## Summary

It is apparent that there are many issues that play therapists need to be mindful of when becoming involved in therapeutic practice with children:

- what self-care really means
- the impact of trauma upon the "caring cycle"
- burnout and compassion fatigue risks

- the challenges and pitfalls of self-care
- professional competence for practice

With this knowledge in mind, we as therapists can begin to grapple with the subjectivity of what may prevent or promote successful self-care in our practical lives and, as stated by Skovholt and Trotter-Mathison (2016: 164), ". . . we must continue self-care but do so at an accelerated pace". Getting it wrong sometimes or trying something out and realising that it does not work for you is okay. This is a skill that we develop alongside our practice, so perhaps there should never come a time when we feel we have conquered self-care, but instead are running parallel to it, changing and adapting. The tools that I have highlighted work for me at this current time, but it is important to acknowledge that if you cannot access your preferred methods or they no longer work for you, it is worth reflecting on whether your needs have changed or the circumstances within which you are working are different.

To summarise my research, I chose to create a poem, called "Breathe", that explored the themes identified throughout and in the spirit of heuristic research and playfulness, and it feels appropriate to share this at the end of this chapter. Do not ignore things, take notice and adapt if it feels right to do so. Do not take my word for it, trust your own instinct, we have it for a reason.

### "Breathe"

Put on your oxygen mask, don't hold your breath,
suffocation by others can cause early death.
The smog, the fumes, the hurt and the pain,
keeps on falling, like acid rain.

Expectations needs and stress,
adds to the burden that begins to press,
hold onto thy self with all your might,
it won't be easy; this will be a fight.

The love of the work that gives us such pleasure,
too much, too soon will find its real measure.
Boundaries and balance, workload, and pace,
all add to the illusion we've entered a race.

The chaos, the confusion, the fuss, and blame,
in the end we all realise this isn't a game.
We search for more meaning and knowledge to master,
but then we feel tricked, it's all a disaster.

From the darkness there comes a small beam,
self-care and self-worth, what does it mean?

Our journey continues for as long as we care,
the light gets brighter the more we stare.

So, what did we learn during our sortie?
That self-care continues long after forty.
The skills need learning and that's what matters,
so, our therapist selves won't end up in tatters.

## References

Baker, E. K. (2003) *Caring for Ourselves: A Therapist's Guide to Personal and Professional Wellbeing*. Washington, DC: American Psychological Association.

Bowlby, J. (1988) *A Secure Base: Clinical Applications of Attachment Theory*. London: Routledge.

British Association of Counselling and Psychotherapists. (2018) *Ethical Framework for the Counselling Professions*. Available at: www.bacp.co.uk/media/3103/bacp-ethical-framework-for-the-counselling-professions-2018.pdf (Accessed: 28 July 2018).

British Association of Play Therapists. (2020) *Ethical Basis for Good Practice in Play Therapy. Updated 2020*. Available at: www.bapt.info/play-therapy/ethical-basis-good-practice-play-therapy/ (Accessed: 17 June 2021).

British Psychoanalytic Council. (2011) *Code of Ethics*. Available at: www.bpc.org.uk/sites/psychoanalytic-council.org/files/4.1%20Code%20of%20Ethics%20Feb%202011.pdf (Accessed: 2 April 2018).

Brownn, E. (2013) *My Spiritual Sabbatical*. Available at: https://eleanorbrownn.wordpress.com/page/4/ (Accessed: 29 October 2017).

Centre for Personal & Professional Development Counselling School. (2017) Self-Care: How Do You Take Care of Yourself? *Therapy Today: The Voice of the Counselling and Psychotherapy Profession*, 28(7), p. 44.

Cochran, N. H., Nordling, W. J. & Cochran, J. L. (2010) *Child-Centered Play Therapy: A Practical Guide to Developing Therapeutic Relationships With Children*. Hoboken, NJ: John Wiley & Sons.

Davis Bush, A. (2015) *Simple Self Care for Therapists: Restorative Practices to Weave Through Your Workday*. New York: W.W. Norton and Company.

Figley, C. R. (1995) Compassion Fatigue: Toward a New Understanding of the Costs of Caring. In: Stamm, B. H. (ed.) *Secondary Traumatic Stress: Self-Care Issues for Clinicians, Researchers and Educators* (pp. 3–28). Baltimore: Sidran Press.

Freudenberger, H. J. (1975) The Staff Burn-Out Syndrome in Alternative Institutions. *Psychotherapy: Theory, Research, and Practice*, 12(1), pp. 73–82.

Landreth, G. L. (2012) *Play Therapy: The Art of the Relationship* (3rd ed.). New York: Routledge.

Maschi, T. (2015) Professional Self-Care and the Prevention of Secondary Trauma Among Play Therapists Working With Traumatised Youth. In: Boyd-Webb, N. (ed.) *Play Therapy With Children and Adolescents in Crisis* (4th ed, pp. 395–416). New York: Guilford Press.

Meany-Walen, K. K., Cobie-Nuss, A., Eittreim, E., Teeling, S., Wilson, S. & Xander, C. (2018) Play Therapists' Perceptions of Wellness and Self-Care Practices. *International Journal of Play Therapy*, 27(3), pp. 176–186.

Moustakas, C. (1990) *Heuristic Research: Design, Methodology, and Applications*. London: Sage Publications.

Oxford University Press (2017) *Oxford Dictionary*. Available at: https://en.oxforddic tionaries.com/definition/self-care (Accessed: 4 November 2017).

Parsons, R. D. & Zhang, N. (2014) *Becoming a Skilled Counsellor*. Thousand Oaks, CA: Sage Publications.

Play Therapy United Kingdom. (2013) *Ethical Framework for Play Therapy and Filial Play and Professional Conduct Procedure Ethical Framework for Play Therapy and Filial Play*. Available at: www.playtherapy.org/Portals/0/documents/PTUKEthics2010V3_31. pdf?ver=2016-10-27-121446-767.

Ray, D. C. (2011) *Advanced Play Therapy: Essential Conditions, Knowledge, and Skills for Child Practice*. New York: Routledge.

Rogers, C. R. (1951) *Client-Centred Therapy*. London: Constable.

Rogers, C. R. (1980) *A Way of Being*. New York: Houghton Mifflin.

Rothschild, B. & Rand, M. (2006) *Help for the Helper: The Psychophysiology of Compassion Fatigue and Vicarious Trauma*. New York: W. W. Norton & Company.

Selye, H. (1974) *Stress Without Distress*. London: Hodder and Stoughton Ltd.

Skovholt, T. M. (2005) The Cycle of Caring: A Model of Expertise in the Helping Professions. *Journal of Mental Health Counselling*, 27(1), pp. 82–94.

Skovholt, T. M. & Trotter-Mathison, M. (2016) *The Resilient Practitioner: Burnout and Compassion Fatigue Prevention and Self-Care Strategies for the Helping Professions*. (3rd ed.). London: Routledge.

Shapiro, F. (2007) EMDR, Adaptive Information Processing, and Case Conceptualization. *Journal of EMDR Practice and Research*, 1(2), pp. 68–87.

United Kingdom Council for Psychotherapy. (2009) *Ethical Principles and Code of Professional Conduct*. Available at: www.psychotherapy.org.uk/wp-content/uploads/2017/11/ UKCP-Ethical-Principles-and-Code-of-Professional-Conduct.pdf (Accessed: 2 April 2018).

Wilkins, P. (2016) *Person-Centered Therapy: 100 Key Points and Techniques* (2nd ed.). Oxon: Routledge.

Woodward-Myers, T. & Cornille, T. A. (2002) The Trauma of Working With Traumatised Children. In: Figley, C. R. (ed.) *Treating Compassion Fatigue* (pp. 39–55). New York: Brunner-Routledge.

# Chapter 10

# The art of witnessing

## Exploring the interplay between play therapy, theatre and supervision

*Ann Marie John*

### Setting the scene

As play therapists, we interweave our professional and personal lives in a manner that is unique to the therapeutic profession. We cannot keep them completely separate, nor is it helpful or desirable to do so, although we do need to maintain professional boundaries. Existential therapists such as Patrick Casement (2013) have helpfully documented that not only do we influence our clients, but they also in turn influence us. We use supervision and personal therapy as a space to reflect upon this process of mutual influence. We try to work out which emotions are ours and which are our clients' and how can we both move forward together. At times, events in our family life cycle – births, deaths, separations and other life experiences – may both challenge and compliment this process. This chapter aims to describe how I have found my own way of exploring the space between the personal and the professional, a way which I find enhances my practice, keeps it safe and prevents burnout and secondary trauma. I hope that it will encourage you to find your own means of renewal and to think, reflect and write about this process.

In preparing to write this chapter, curiosity led me to look up the origins and meanings of the word *process*. The Cambridge English Dictionary (2020) defines *process* as a "series of actions that you take in order to achieve a result" or a "series of changes that happen naturally". The Online Etymology Dictionary (2020) describes the word's origin as coming from the medieval French, translated as "the fact of being carried on" or as I prefer, a "going forward, advance progress". I particularly like the term "going forward" as this seems pertinent to the intention within our professional practice. We may not know where we are going but we aim to go forward. In this chapter then, I reflect on how witnessing live theatre has helped me with "a going forward" in my process of witnessing and working with the stories of my clients and their families.

### Act one, scene one: process in the play therapy room

Play therapy process, I would argue, is a developmental process or a series of processes. It is a going forward for both the therapist and the young person and

DOI: 10.4324/9781003017271-10

indeed their families. The experience of play therapy feeds back into the child's organic systems, into the body, brain and nervous system and equally into the play therapist's own neurobiological system. Further to this, I would suggest there are a number of interrelating processes in play therapy, all of which help organise meaning and experience for the child and indeed for the therapist. We are often changed by our experiences in the playroom.

The process I wish to explore within this chapter is that of "witnessing" and in particular witnessing the emotional expression of the child. I have found Schon's (2016) ideas about learning and development very helpful in terms of thinking about witnessing. Schon refers to the process of reflecting not only on action (as we do in clinical supervision) but also *in action* as we respond to the child in the moment, adapting and changing. We have a rationale for our responses in the play therapy room, even if sometimes we seem to be "doing" very little and are staying with the not knowing. Witnessing is not therefore passive; it is active and intentional. Schon writes about the development of "on action" to "in action" (2016: 105) so that our reflections become active therapeutic interventions within the session. I find this a particularly helpful idea when thinking about how the practice of witnessing develops during the course of the therapeutic process.

## Act one, scene two: interrelating contexts and parallel processes

One of the ways that helps me to monitor my responses to the child is to think about distance and connection. What is my response to the child's emotional expression? How close or distanced do I feel? Am I avoiding or overidentifying with the child's feelings? How do I manage the metaphorical and sometimes very real mess in the room whilst maintaining my own emotional regulation and equilibrium? One suggestion in helping to manage these therapeutic challenges is to engage in creative parallel processes. Whilst my chosen process is the experience of witnessing live theatre, there are also other experiences I will sometimes engage with that help my capacity to process and stay with the often-uncomfortable feelings engendered by the work.

A recent example of this is from my experience of a pottery throwing course. I recall feeling profound frustration with the wheel as I struggled to make progress with my work. I also did not enjoy the messiness of the clay and the effort of constantly clearing my wheel and starting again. However, I realised a few days later that something had shifted for me psychologically and although the course had not felt that productive for me in terms of output or skill development, the process of engaging with all the mess was invaluable to me personally in terms of re-connecting me with the therapeutic value of wading through the "mess" of the work. These kinds of creative, parallel processes can, I would suggest, allow us to stay with that liminal space that lies between the processes of *reflecting on* and *being in action with,* a space that enables the therapeutic process to keep moving.

The premise of this chapter then is to explore how personal processes of renewal can help us with both "reflection in action" and "on action" in the play therapy process. While different therapists may have different processes of reflection, my own relates to my experiences (and passion) for live theatre and in particular Greek Tragedy. I suggest that the experience of witnessing theatre helps me in the process of witnessing emotion in play therapy and the way I reflect in the moment in the play room.

## Act two, scene one: the main focus

The act of witnessing the dramatic worlds of characters within a play, at a distance, helps me to connect with my own emotional process in a similar way to how play therapy enables the child to play out their feelings in an emotionally distanced way. It helps to regulate and re-organise my emotional responses and facilitate a healthy return to the playroom and to reflect on my feelings and actions.

Throughout the course of my career, going to the theatre has helped me to connect with deep emotions, which in turn have enabled me to create more meaningful relational contexts with the children and families I am working with. I suggest then that the heightened emotional nature of theatre performance aligns with the therapy process, creating the possibility for rites of passage and renewal, helping me connect with the interface between the personal and professional. I will now begin to give some examples of how these two processes interrelate, sharing experiences from my career.

## Act two, scene two: the play and playing

The first "proper" play I saw was Oedipus Rex by Sophocles (1984) at the Manchester Exchange Theatre at the age of 19. I had never experienced anything like it. As well as being moved to tears, I felt that the witnessing of the extreme emotion of the play (with Oedipus realising the terrible truth that he had inadvertently married his mother and killed his father) left me with a profound sense of reconnecting with what it means to be human. It was only several years later while training as a dramatherapist that I discovered the term "catharsis", a kind of emotional cleansing that Aristotle wrote about when analysing the process and function of Greek drama in his book The Poetics (2013). Tierno (2002: 98) applying Aristotle's principles to screen writing, comments that the "combination of physical suffering and emotional suffering helps intensify the emotions of the audience, who feeling the tragedy in their very bones are swept away".

I strongly relate to that feeling, of my bones being swept away, and whilst Tierno writes that a process of catharsis can be experienced through cinema, I would argue that the live witnessing of theatre is more powerful because the emotional witnessing of the drama is a direct feedback loop between audience and actors, in constant non-verbal dialogue with each other. This is similar to the process of play therapy. No two nights at the theatre are the same, and no two play therapy sessions are the same. Tierno writing on Aristotle argues that "catharsis leaves the audience with a renewed sense of mental clarity and better able to function in life" (2016: 98). I could not put it better myself.

Since that first experience, I have continually sought out similar cathartic experiences. Now having studied theatre and the classics further, I realise that Oedipus Rex is often referred to as a perfect play in terms of its plotting and the way the story and the characters position the audience. We are aware of Oedipus's mistake in trying to avoid the fateful prophecy and that ultimately, his attempt to escape his fate ends in tragic failure.

This witnessing of distress is both similar to play therapy and different in that it touches our deepest fears whilst we know it not to be real. The play therapy process is also about pretence and reality. The child's feelings are no less real because they are expressed through play. The feelings we experience as an audience in response to a play are no less real because we suspend our disbelief. While the playroom and the therapeutic boundaries keep the child's emotional world safe, the process of dramatic play facilitates emotional distance and makes our witnessing (and that of the child's) bearable. In the playroom, as on the stage, the child has the opportunity to express feelings intensely. This might be through role-play or projective play but also perhaps something more embodied and sensory; a child emptying a whole tube of paint onto the paper and revelling in both the mess and the permission to create it.

In my play therapy career, I have become very adept at hamming up my character's death as a witch, neglectful parent or general all-round baddie. During one sword fight, my death went on for some time as I cried out in ever-increasing pain and the child asked me to repeat the performance again and again, much to his delight and excitement. In this situation, I both witness and amplify the child's emotion in the safety of the play. We are pretending and no one is hurt. In parallel, when I am at the theatre, the intensity of the emotion feels real, but I know at another level that it is not. I suspend my disbelief. I suggest that this enables me to process some of the feelings I might feel in the playroom.

## Act three, scene one

"Meaning making" or making sense of a child's experience is an important element of play therapy. I think this can often be overlooked, as during the course of the therapeutic process, there is a constant re-storying and re-authoring of experience to help make sense of it. I suggest there is also a parallel with the therapist's process and we need to be particularly aware of this when our personal lives are challenging. After my mother's recent funeral, I drove my daughter back to university where she was directing a production of Antigone, another of my favourite Greek plays by Sophocles, in which the stakes are high. I had intended to drive home but felt too tired and decided to stay over. I also decided I may as well go to see the play. While the logic of going to the theatre might seem strange, after a funeral, I realised that it made sense in my family. My mother would have not wanted my daughter to miss her production and I felt my mother's presence throughout. I recognised the familiar words of the play and once again witnessed the titular character's inevitable downfall as she insists on giving her brother customary burial rites despite the fact that it has been decreed that this is against the law and punishable by death. I drove home the following day feeling that I was ready to return to work and if I had not seen the play, I am not sure that I would have been so ready. Tierno (2002) suggests that the final catharsis of witnessing the protagonist's suffering helps us to both learn about life's meaning and face our darker side, and ultimately our own death.

## Act three, scene two: theatre as emotional regulation. Avoiding burnout and re-traumatisation

As therapists working with trauma, we are faced with emotional dysregulation on a daily basis. Whilst within the therapeutic process this can be managed safely, it does not mean that we are not affected and can experience secondary traumatisation (Stamm, 1995). A child kills me repeatedly with an imaginary gun, expressing his intense feelings of anger and rage, redirected towards me. No doubt, we have all come out of sessions like this feeling emotionally overwhelmed, distressed or simply exhausted. Those of us working with young people experience the expression of trauma and dysregulation through their self-harming and suicidal behaviour, and family members can express it through their blaming and shaming, often expressed directly towards us as professionals. Sometimes we notice our colleagues and ourselves becoming dysregulated and we hopefully seek and are sought after for support. Supervision and personal therapy can help us with this.

Characters within theatre also dysregulate at times, and interpersonal conflict is the central premise of dramatic performance. When I see a play, I also witness trauma, and the fact that I must suspend my disbelief (I know it is not real but is true in the moment) also makes it safe, through the process of role and aesthetic distance. The witnessing of trauma and dysregulation in a play enables me to reflect on action and my own therapeutic practice within the playroom. Within dramatic performance, conflict is also often bordered by comedy and I can experience sadness and laughter together (pathos). Safely witnessing the performance of such conflictual and disparate emotions often helps me to feel more regulated and better able to manage the intense emotions that I am exposed to in my work on a daily basis.

The following example illustrates a day in my practice when things were tough going. I am in a meeting in my role as family therapist in an in-patient mental health unit and decide, perhaps foolishly, to challenge a father regarding his criticism that we have done nothing to help his daughter after six months in hospital. His daughter's mental health is actually much better from the professional point of view. Against my better judgement, I decided to challenge him about his critical approach, which I think mirrors the way he behaves to his daughter. I know this father well and when he feels vulnerable, he often becomes verbally aggressive and attacking. I know he does this to his family and to his daughter who also dysregulates emotionally, but I feel the need to defend my team. I challenge him about the service and the fact he has not attended the training we provide for parents. He targets me personally and complains that I have not given them strategies for coping and tells me the whole family agree about how unhelpful I have been.

Things have to be decided and the meeting moves on, but I am unusually shaken and am tearful for most of the afternoon. My ward doctor kindly supports me and I leave to go to my other professional role, training family therapists, and the change of context within which I feel more an expert and perhaps in control is helpful. I also attend a training event and although I am fragile, I can hide how upset I am feeling. I am angry with myself for walking into such an escalation, and it is a long time since I have felt this upset at work. It was a very public humiliation and I try to identify with the daughter and what it must be like for her, but it is a struggle.

Fortunately, that evening I go to a new play by my favourite modern playwright, Carol Churchill (2019), which consists of four short pieces. The first is a surreal story about China figures on a mantlepiece that are alive. Then in the second, Bluebeard's friends discuss their dilemmas about him at a dinner party, not knowing that he is in fact a serial killer. In the third, a Greek god sitting on a cloud recounts tales from Greek mythology and the traumatic experiences of humans, their dysfunctional families and horrific stories of murder and sacrifice. The final chorus in this piece is particularly powerful as we hear the words "stop it" repeated again and again. The final play of the quartet is my favourite, about two older and rather sad characters, living on benefits, sitting in their lounge telling stories to each other. One tells the story of the magic imp she believes lives in a bottle whilst the other, her cousin, retells Shakespeare's tragedies but in the context of the man down the pub who is having a hard time with his daughters (King Lear). I get texts of support from my colleagues at work about what happened in the meeting. My friend buys me the play script and I smile for almost the first time that day. I am all right, the tearfulness has gone and something has lifted.

Back at work the next day, I am able to acknowledge that my intervention in the meeting might have been unhelpful. I was able to adopt my usual stance of putting myself in the position of the parent, having to manage the worry (and shame) of your child being in an adolescent unit. I am back to a position where my work is my bread and butter and not my nemesis. I have witnessed others on stage battling their own personal demons and I am now back in a space where I have regained some balance and neutrality. When I reflect on this now, I recognise my own over-identification with the young daughter and that perhaps I was trying to rescue her, something that happens to all of us at various points in our practice.

## Act four, therapy as performance: shoulds, oughts and imposter syndrome – a sub-plot

Staying with the dramatic metaphor for a while, I am interested in the idea of how life roles are performed rather than the significance of a role itself. Performance is a part of being a therapist and whilst we have scripts to ensure that we address important areas of practice, for example contracts, confidentiality and assessments, we are also free to improvise around these scripts. I find that witnessing live theatre helps me to reflect upon the process of my therapeutic practice and of the "performance" of my various professional roles. As part of this reflective process, I suggest that there is a certain moral aspect to our work, which I like to think of as "shoulds and oughts". For example, how much mess should we allow the child to make before they feel too uncontained? When do we need to put a boundary in? Our training, supervision and continuing professional development all contribute to this and in a sense we become a critical audience to ourselves and our own practice. Sometimes we might also get anxious before a session and I know that many of my colleagues experience a sense of "imposter syndrome", wherein at certain times in a session, we feel that we are unworthy of the work we do and feel like a fraud that one day might be found out. Given that this experience seems so common among therapists I feel it must serve some kind of useful function. Indeed, it is often when I am feeling my most confident that I am struck by this sudden experience of self-doubt. I might be passionately arguing my case with a psychiatrist or giving parenting advice when I ask myself "what on earth makes me have the audacity to act in this way"?

I suggest that theatre helps me with this performance of my professional self and to sit more comfortably with being a critical audience to myself and to make friends with my imposter syndrome. I see it as a break in performance. It is like the role of the chorus in the Greek tragedies in commenting on the action or a Brechtian play when the actor moves out of role to talk to the audience. It can also be important to question one's performance and in this sense perhaps imposter syndrome helps to maintain a degree of humility, reminding us that our performance is for the client and not for ourselves. Of course, imposter syndrome can also be very negative and cripple our self-confidence, although I believe that being honest and open about our feelings can help make this experience our friend rather than our foe.

## Act five, scene one

Over-identification, or over-distancing as a form of dysregulation, is another emotional coping strategy that can be unhelpful. By over-distancing, I am meaning a sense of becoming too distanced from the client and feeling disconnected or uncaring. I acknowledge that I have sometimes experienced client's problems as trivial, more so in my private practice compared to the acute, complex nature of my NHS or local authority work. But this is not my usual position and having talked with colleagues, I know that I am not alone in this occasional experience of over-distancing myself from my work. When my colleague's partner and my own partner were both diagnosed with cancer, we admitted to both feeling that at times we wanted to tell clients to "get on with it". Yet this is not the only outcome of experiencing difficult, personal life-cycle issues. There have been many times when I have felt most connected to my clients and indeed most helpful to them when I have been going through a challenging experience myself. That said, sometimes things have felt a little too close to home.

I think this distancing, lack of connection or caring less about the client can have a number of elements contributing to it but I do think it is a sign or a need for renewal. This could be through supervision or continuing professional development (CPD) but I increasingly access the theatre for support, where I feel reconnected with my capacity to care deeply. I find this an incredibly healthy experience – something that helps me safely manage both risk and the kind of deeply intense emotion that I might otherwise choose to avoid.

## Act five, scene two: the theatre of supervision

Recently, I went to see "The Greek Play" at the University of Cambridge, a play performed every two years, in ancient Greek (with subtitles), in connection with the university's classics department. The play was Oedipus at Colonus, not one I know so well and not so often performed. It was stunning in every sense, from the wonderful chants of the chorus to the rhythm of the Greek language, re-claiming the story and characters as they deal with the will of the gods.

What I was particularly stuck by in this play was the impact of the chorus and its role as a reflective process. As well as the beauty of the singing, the commentary on the action and sometimes the wise words to the main character, the chorus struck me as a voice of reason, perhaps not dissimilar to the process of clinical supervision. I realised that this witnessing of the chorus was connecting me to something of my own experience both as a supervisee and as a supervisor, and to my surprise, I found that SparkNotes (an online study guide) provided a description of the role of the chorus that connected with my sense of a parallel process at play. "The chorus reacts to events as they happen, generally in a predictable, though not consistent, way. It generally expresses a longing for calm and stability" (SparkNotes, 2020).

Whilst having authority, the chorus in Greek tragedy is on the whole a non-judgemental voice and is usually performed by a group, so has a feeling of democracy as it reflects externally on the action. In many ways, these are the essential qualities of a clinical supervisor in facilitating a practitioner to safely reflect upon their work. However, in the same way that supervision might also gently challenge the supervisee, the chorus might reflect and comment on the main character's position.

At the end of Antigone, when Creon realises he has in fact gone against the wishes of the gods, the chorus chants Seamus Heaney's translation:

Wise conduct is the key to happiness.
Always rule by the gods and reverence them.

> Those who overbear will be brought to grief.
> Fate will flail them on its winnowing floor
> And in due season teach them to wise.
>
> (2004: 74)

Heaney's (2004) translation is poetic rather than literal and whilst play therapy supervision does not necessarily take us to the dramatic heights of Greek tragedy, it does involve reflecting on the moral and ethical dilemmas of our practice as therapists. Within the supervision process, the supervisor witnesses the emotional life of the therapist. As supervisors we are, I suggest helping the therapist to create a relationship between the "shoulds and oughts" of their ethical positioning. Sometimes we comment on the nature of the stories they bring to supervision and, in a similar way to the chorus, we pay attention to our supervisees emotional state, as they do to their clients. Our supervisors inform, commentate and advise upon our practice, in a sense both judging and not judging, similar to that of the role of the chorus.

We contract with our supervisees to enable them to acknowledge feelings of vulnerability, whilst also offering a degree of constructive challenge that supports their practice and ensures that we are both working in the best interests of the client. My thinking on this has perhaps changed over the years, having reflected upon what it means to be non-judgemental, or indeed judgemental. By judgemental, I do not mean shaming or insisting that there is a right or wrong way to do something, but more a gentle taking of different positions that allows me sometimes to be open, honest and direct if I need to challenge, and be challenged. The position of supervisory frankness is something that has also developed as part of my developing clinical practice and I will have a conversation with parents at the start of therapy to explain that I will be open and honest with them if I need to be. In the most part, they value and appreciate this approach, and this process of creating a context for openness is also part of the supervision contract when we have a conversation about the need to challenge.

I also find it useful to have these conversations with myself when I am undertaking individual play therapy and I find the idea of the Greek chorus helps me to prepare for and process sessions. Perhaps having the experience of being a systemic family therapy supervisor, observing from behind a screen and intervening through reflective conversations that the family are a part of, has helped me internalise ways of accessing other voices in my work.

I recall a recent session in which I was witnessing a child's play in the sand. My internalised "chorus" commented that "the child makes circles in the sand and I am watching and mirroring his body language". The word circle felt very significant and I started very gently to make some circular movements with my hand, an echo of the child's play in the sand. The child looked up at me and made eye contact and I wanted to draw circles in the sand too. The child's eye contact felt important but it did not feel like an invitation to join. My internalised dialogue and the small circular movements of my hand had helped me to judge my next move, and it was through witnessing the child's play and my own subsequent actions in response to his play that I realised my urge to join in was more my need than his. This critical, internalised witnessing of my own "performance" also required a holding on to both the judgemental and non-judgemental voices, which connects back to previously discussed imposter syndrome and the "shoulds and oughts" of my inner chorus.

At the end of Antigone, Creon acknowledges his folly that in refusing to allow Polynices his burial rights, he has gone against the gods. The Chorus and Creon have a dialogue:

> Creon: Let every verdict be pronounced
> Against me. She was guiltless.
> It was my hand on the hilt,
> My hand on that drive the blade.
> Take me out of your sight
> I am nothing now.
> Forget me. Treat me as nothing.
>
> The Chorus Answer:
> This is right, but if right can very come
> From wrongs like ours. This is good
> When the worst has to be faced, the best thing is to face it quickly.
>
> (2004: 72)

These words for me communicate something of the benevolent duality of the supervisory process, to simultaneously both judge and not judge, a position that I seek to hold in relation to both my own self-supervision and my supervision of others. Of course, the voice of the chorus can be intense and harsh. When I see and hear the chorus on stage, the dramatic stakes are always high, mere mortals making life-or-death decisions against the will of the gods. But then the stakes are also high in therapy, as we hold the clinical responsibility of working with young people and always having to keep issues of safeguarding and risk in mind. My experience of witnessing and hearing the chorus is one of a supporting voice that somehow helps me to reflect upon and contain the responsibilities I hold as a supervisor and therapist.

## Act five, scene three: final thoughts from the chorus

In this chapter then, I hope to have shared something about how witnessing theatre, and in particular Greek theatre, has helped me to be able to think deeply about the significance of witnessing in therapy. Further to this is the support it provides in helping me regulate my emotions and avoid secondary trauma and burnout and to think about the position I take in supervision. Whilst writing this, during the pandemic, going to the theatre has not been possible, which has been something of a personal challenge, but in times ahead I would recommend Greek theatre, or indeed any type of theatre, as a way of helping to manage both our professional practice as therapists and the more personal experience of stages of the life cycle.

## References

Aristotle (trans. Anthony, K. 2013) *Poetics* (Reprint ed.). Oxford: Oxford University Press.

Cambridge English Dictionary (2020) Available at: https://dictionary.cambridge.org/dictionary/english/ (Accessed: 20 November 2020).

Casement, C. (2013) *On Learning from the Patient* (2nd ed.). London: Routledge.

Churchill, C. (2019) *Glass. Kill. Bluebeard. Imp* (Play Script). London: Nick Hern Books.

Heaney, S. (2004) *The Burial at Thebes Sophocles Antigone*. London: Faber and Faber.

Online Etymology Dictionary. (2020) Available at: www.etymonline.com/ (Accessed: 20 November 2020).

Schon, D. A. (2016) *The Reflective Practitioner: How Professionals Think in Action*. London: Routledge.

Sophocles (trans. Knox, B. 1984) *The Three Theban Plays: 'Antigone', 'Oedipus the King', 'Oedipus at Colonus'*. London: Penguin Classics.

SparkNotes. (2020) Available at: www.sparknotes.com/drama/oedipus/character/the-chorus/ (Accessed: 20 November 2020).

Stamm, B. H. (ed.). (1995) *Secondary Traumatic Stress: Self-Care Issues for Clinicians, Researchers, and Educators*. Baltimore: The Sidran Press.

Tierno. (2002) *Aristotle's Poetics for Screenwriters: Storytelling Secrets From the Greatest Mind in Western Civilisations*. New York: Hyperion.

# Chapter 11

# Tremor

## Shaken and stirred

*David Le Vay*

The consultant sat us down and tore out a bit of paper from his notepad and started drawing a rudimentary sketch: A couple of small circles, a dot here and there and an arrow or two suggesting movement of some sort. It could have been the solar system, planets in orbit around the sun and arrows indicating gravitational force. Or it could have been an atom, electrons spinning giddily around a central nucleus. But somehow, I did not think a neurology consultant would be concerning himself with astronomy or particle physics. I recall wondering to myself how often he had drawn this little sketch, my breath held in a frozen moment of time. He looked up from his drawing and held eye contact, steady and sure. I fought the urge to look away, flinching, as if to try and dodge the anticipated bullet, but his aim was true.

"So" he said calmly, "this is what we call Parkinson's".

In unison, as if choreographed, my partner and I exhaled sharply, as if the oxygen had been sucked from our lungs by some kind of invisible force. A punch in the gut left us momentarily breathless. Who knew simple words could have such force? The consultant explained his drawing; the neurons, neurotransmitters, the arrows indicating the directional flow of dopamine, or the absence of, in my case. But I was only half listening at this point, my cognitive processing capacity temporarily hijacked by other, more primitive systems. There was an incongruity about the consultant's calmness; I wanted to scream, protest, cry, shout, deny, escape, hide. Instead, I simply sat and nodded, as if being given directions to the nearest supermarket. Latterly, I have thought about this in the context of our work as play therapists, as we listen to and observe children's stories of loss, abuse and trauma. Maybe we should shout a little louder – "that's not fair, it shouldn't have happened to you!". As a young, protesting child my father always used to tell me that life is unfair. Well, now I know he was right.

I was diagnosed in October 2019, two months before my partner and I were due to leave for a long planned for, six-month travelling adventure to New Zealand, Australia and the Greek Islands. It was to be a once in a lifetime trip, and the consultant said there was no reason not to go, and so we did. Two months later, we found ourselves on an anxious, hastily booked flight back from New Zealand to the United Kingdom, face masks on and flying headlong into the epicentre of

DOI: 10.4324/9781003017271-11

a global pandemic. I am not religious, far from it, but it certainly felt like something or someone was conspiring against us. It was not quite the adventure we had planned. All this at the same time as writing and editing a book on personal process within child-centred play therapy, and whilst the fantasy was that I would be spending the days tapping away on my laptop in a chilled-out bar on a Greek island, beside the sunlit, warm, cerulean-blue waters of the Mediterranean, the reality proved to be very different. I had not quite anticipated that I would have this much "personal process" to deal with.

In a strange way, the pandemic provided the perfect cover for my Parkinson's diagnosis. I could legitimately hide away from the world; hide the shame and stigma that I felt so acutely through having my neurological fault lines so visibly exposed. I felt the urge – the need – to retreat from society and so the prescribed pandemic principles of social distance, isolation and quarantine came very easily. But like any retreat, it came at a cost and alongside my family, I was forcefully required to re-evaluate the future and what lay ahead. What did this mean in terms of my personal and professional identity, my role as a partner, father, play therapist, lecturer? I slipped into talking about myself in the past tense – the "used to" man. I used to play the piano, I used to run, I used to hike, I used to teach, I used to be a therapist. Maybe I will continue to do all, some or none of these things, who knows, but the label, like the condition itself, began to enclose me; insidious, unforgiving, unrelenting . . . holding me tight in its tremulous grip whilst outside, the Covid storm raged on, providing an intense, traumatic global counterpoint to my own, very personal, existential crisis.

To reflect upon and write about my personal process as a play therapist during this period has, to the say the least, been something of a challenge and my decision to write this chapter comes as a response to this challenge. Like the incongruence of my consultant's calm voice as he delivered his devastating news, it would feel incongruent, within a book of this nature, not to write about my own personal process during this period of time and of the ongoing impact of both my diagnosis and the Covid pandemic. Indeed, the two have become somewhat intertwined. And also, perhaps, I write this chapter as a way of "coming out", to claim the label before it claims me; to try and hold my gaze and stare it down. Quite how helpful this process will be, time will tell; the jury is still out, so to speak. Certainly, in the early days of my diagnosis, I found myself caught within a relentless and psychologically exhausting conflict between acceptance and denial, the inevitable truth slowly but surely taking shape, just as a sculptor gradually reveals a recognisable form from a block of granite, relentlessly chipping away at the unyielding, resistant stone. Beaten, hammered and chiselled, my capacity for pretence was slowly worn down and the truth revealed. Over the course of the first year, I told no one about my situation, beyond my immediate family and a few close work colleagues, and it is only more recently that I have begun to share it more openly. And of course, the Covid pandemic colluded in this secrecy, allowing me to hide, locked down, in plain sight, the embodied nature of the disease being sanitised and cleansed, like the virus, by the disembodied frame of the zoom screen. Not a tremor in sight.

My aim then, within this chapter, is to explore from both professional and personal perspectives the impact of my diagnosis, within the wider context of the COVID-19 pandemic. How have these twin challenges affected my practice as a play therapist and my role as a Senior Lecturer on an MA Play Therapy programme? What are the wider implications of therapist illness and how we manage this? What are some of the longer term implications for play therapy as we are forced as a profession to adapt and find new ways of working with children? What are the challenges and the opportunities? And what has been the experience of editing a book on personal process in the midst of this storm? Of course, there may be no answers, no certainty, just more questions. As I write this, in April 2021, the United Kingdom begins to cautiously emerge, blinking and inoculated into the warming spring sunshine after a year of intermittent lockdown. But beyond our shores, the pandemic rages on and I suspect that there will be a few more plot twists along the way.

## On loss and longing

Perhaps the greatest emotional impact of my diagnosis has been around the intense experience of loss, or more to the point, the anticipation of loss. I am left grieving for a future not yet lived. I mourn a sense of lost possibility. As my condition "progresses" (an odd misnomer of the Parkinson's lexicon), I find myself having to let go of little parts of myself; faded, perfumed petals of vitality snatched away by the bitter wind and carried away into the recent past, leaving behind just the forlorn shape of a memory. As the author Julian Barnes says in Levels of Life, his seminal book on grief and loss – "what happiness is there in just the memory of happiness?" (2014: 79).

As I lose the movement and dexterity of my left hand, I can no longer play percussion and my collection of North African drums lies on the shelf, silent and untouched. I can no longer tap out a simple rhythm on the steering wheel of my car as I sit waiting for the lights to change (a rare bonus, my partner might say). My ability to play the piano is diminished, and I lose both enjoyment and confidence in the process. The disembodied, unintegrated impact of Parkinson's means that I have lost an intuitive sense of my inner musicality, the soundtrack to my life. This is devastating beyond words and I can only hope that it is something that I can find again. I will probably have to call time on the band that I have been playing with for the last seven years – my other family. Having played in bands all my adult life, is this another thing I will have to let go? I can still just about manage a very short run but my regular routine of tough 10 km runs and half marathons is a thing of the past. And as for my penchant for long distance hiking, who knows. Having in my time walked coast to coast along the entire length of the French Pyrenees, hiked around Mont Blanc, sweated across the mountains of Mallorca, run around Menorca and slipped, slid and scrambled across the rugged interior of Corsica, walking has been an intrinsic part of my life and identity. My last long-distance hike was along the Atlantic coast of Portugal, the famed

Fisherman's Trail, in the delightful company of my daughter. It was a truly special experience. It might also prove to be my last. Now I walk with a disguised limp, flat-footed and awkward, my left leg failing to do what my right brain is telling it to do. I feel like an ill-controlled, unrepairable marionette, my strings tangled and frayed, as I wait, helpless, for the next one to snap. At the time of writing, I have – more in hope than expectation – agreed to hike 75 miles along the Cumbria Way in the Lake District with some good friends. I am doubtful as to the outcome: watch this space.

As Woskett (1999: 205) says of therapists,

> [I]f we go through enough loss that belongs to another, we may come to bear our own losses, even the great and final one of our own mortality, more tolerably. If I can bear the pain of this person's anguish and stay with it, enormous as it is, I will be better equipped to bear my own.

In this sense, Woskett goes on to suggest (and with an unknowing nod to the current pandemic) that the "wounded healer may be attempting to immunise themselves against further injury" (1999: 205). But can we really inoculate ourselves from our own emotional pain by dosing ourselves up on that of our clients? What if our own loss becomes too great to bear, struck down by a hitherto unanticipated emotional variant unresponsive to the vicarious client vaccine? Certainly, it has felt too much at times and over the past year I have felt so engulfed by my own pain and loss that I have questioned my capacity to continue my work as a therapist, my confidence dealt a potentially lethal blow by the twin-attack of disease and virus. Indeed, I shocked myself by saying this out loud to my partner – "I don't think I can do this anymore" – and to be fair, she was just as shocked to hear it, shocked that I might be prepared to turn my back on nearly 30 years of clinical practice. But as Guggenbuhl-Craig (1979: 57) suggests, it is only the therapist who is "passionately engaged in their own life who can help his (clients) to find theirs" and I found myself having to question whether I am able to sufficiently balance my own emotional needs with that of my clients, so as to ensure that they do not threaten to overwhelm the therapeutic process.

To be a therapist demands, by definition, a degree of emotional resilience and robustness as we seek to hold, manage and contain the intense distress of our clients. How, then, can I tolerate and contain the pain of the children and families that I am working with if I can barely tolerate my own? What are my moral and ethical responsibilities? What about fitness to practice? Wilton (2001: 1) states that in order to work as a psychotherapist, it is the "responsibility of each of us to make sure we are in a fit state to do so. We must be sound enough physically and emotionally, grounded enough to be able to meet whatever our patients need to bring to us, throw at us, engage us in disentangling". Similar to Wilton's personal account of the impact of illness, I found myself buckling under the existential threat of my Parkinson's, and having to grapple with the uncertainty that I would be able to "continue to fulfil the above pre-requisite" (Wilton, 2001: 1). With my diagnosis coming just before a six-month career break, in conjunction with the pandemic, I had time enough to consider these questions and to reflect upon the longer term implications of my therapeutic work. As it was, I had wound down my caseload prior to my career break and indeed it was not until a year after my initial diagnosis that I made some tentative, small steps back into clinical practice. But along with the personal implications, it was the loss of my professional identity that hit hard, compounding an increasing sense of diminishment.

And with loss comes longing, a deep felt feeling of need – a yearning sense of desire – for what I no longer have and I have had to work hard at this not tipping into self-destructive envy as I know this will only destroy me. I look at people my age as they walk by, longing to be able to move with their physically unencumbered sense of ease. I look at the joggers and the cyclists, my fleeting hopes left hanging in the wind of their teasing slipstream. I look at the cricket ball on the shelf behind me, such playful kinetic potential lying inert, still and unspent. Once again, I have been bamboozled by an erratic bounce on a poor wicket and been caught deep on the boundary, leaving me with a long limping walk back to the pavilion. As they say in sport, it is the hope that kills you.

Of course, the loss is not mine only, and I have to be careful not to try and possess it (or let it possess me), to the exclusion of others. It impacts my family equally, albeit differently, as our shared family narrative lurches in a new, unexpected direction – a plot twist we had not foreseen. Suddenly, we have to renegotiate our relationships with (and to) each other, and find a path together across a new, uncharted landscape. But it is when I allow myself to think about my family, my partner and daughter, and the impact that Parkinson's has and will continue to have on us all, that I feel the sense of loss, and longing, most intensely. But perhaps alongside the losses there are always gains, and I am eternally grateful for the strength and closeness that my family brings. Like the law of unintended consequences, one outcome of the pandemic and ensuing lockdowns has been the very special, privileged times we have been able to share as a family, when it was most needed.

## On reconnecting and disconnecting

Thoughts of family bring to mind the extent to which, fundamentally, we are pro-social, attachment-orientated and proximity-seeking beings. From an intersubjective perspective it is about the relationship between self and other, as Benjamin (2017) suggests, a pleasurable sense of mutual recognition. Child-centred play therapy is about *presence*; it is a relational, embodied process, informed by the implicit interpersonal qualities of attunement and attachment, on both verbal and non-verbal levels. Within this context, I found myself feeling a little uneasy about what felt to be quite a swift, pragmatic move by many to working online, in the wake of the pandemic. This is not a criticism, by any means, and in fact I found myself quite in awe of those people who demonstrated such clinical dexterity in being able to embrace the moment (and the technology) and find new, creative ways of engaging therapeutically with children and families.

Also, it was an issue of timing, having flown back from New Zealand after two months of blissful Covid ignorance, straight into a national lockdown, I was behind the curve, out of sync with the rest of the country, with no time to prepare or adjust to the new reality we suddenly found ourselves in. My long-planned-for career break had been brought to a sudden, rather brutal close, our escapist bubble well and truly burst as we landed, exhausted and anxious, on the runway of Heathrow airport, headlong into the perfect storm of Covid and Parkinson's (not to mention Trump and Brexit). Having rented out our house, we had nowhere to stay and so our immediate need was finding somewhere to live and to be reunited with our daughter. In the shadow of Maslow (1962), shelter, safety and family became our primary concern. Looking back, I can see now what a strange, surreal, anxious and stealthily traumatic time this was, the three of us holed up in a rental cottage in Sussex, avoiding the news and having matter-of-fact conversations about which one of us was least likely to die by going to the supermarket.

Play therapy was far from my mind in the early days of the pandemic and it was not until some months later that I rather tentatively returned to both my university lecturing role and my clinical work, as a member of a small, community-based team of therapists. While colleagues and members of the wider national and international play therapy community adapted with some verve and versatility to the new online paradigm, adopting teletherapy, remote working and the brave, new world order of various virtual platform protocols, I found myself feeling reticent and resistant to make the transition to this new way of working. Certainly, my confidence had been dealt a considerable blow by health anxieties and concerns on several fronts, and I had to play a troubled game of catch up with software programmes hitherto unknown to me, compounded by my usual Luddite ambivalence around technological change.

But there was something more than that. My unease with, and resistance to, adopting the "new normal" of working online was also rooted in the discomfort of having to move away from the theoretical and conceptual child-centred play therapy model that I knew and felt familiar with, indeed that I had trained in. To suddenly switch to working online with children and families was a paradigm shift I felt both unprepared for and, to be honest, unconvinced by. I found it hard to reposition my interpretation of the online terminology of "virtual" and "remote" as meaning anything other than "unreal" and "distant" and as a play therapist I struggled to get beyond the ethical dilemmas of emotional safety, containment and confidentiality and the clinical dilemma of how to maintain therapeutic *presence*.

That said, I also needed to question how much of this was about personal resistance, stubbornness and my own potential blind spots. The answer, as ever, probably lies somewhere in between, but whilst the transition to online therapy held many advantages and created all kinds of new therapeutic possibilities, from an attachment perspective, there seemed to be potential limitations and as Rajkumar

(2020: 258) suggests, the "use of remote technologies for communication may, to a certain extent, undermine rather than facilitate interpersonal interaction". Furthermore, remote working could be problematic for those people already experiencing a degree of social isolation, compounding an already felt sense of disconnection. Thus, whilst teletherapy might "be of immense benefit in some cases, it may be less efficacious in situations where disturbed attachment, or activation of the 'attachment system' by an external trigger, plays an important role" (2020: 259).

So, in a sense I found myself trying to hold a line, a boundary, an anchor even, within a landscape that had shifted dramatically to the point it was almost unrecognisable and maybe this was as much about my own need for security and structure as it was anything else. But all this said, there was certainly a need for play therapists (and trainees) to find ways to support, manage and contain the children and families they had been working with and whose therapeutic process had been disturbed, disrupted and prematurely curtailed through the imposition of national lockdowns, school closures and home confinement. The word "unprecedented" soon became obsolete as we all, in so many ways, found ourselves working (surviving) on the very edge of our experience, clinging on by our very fingertips to what we knew and trusting in what we did not.

Covid subverted the very essence of our inherent, attachment-orientated nature as the nation, the world, had to suddenly adapt to the post-viral rules of social distancing, self-isolation and quarantine. Fear of infection and enforced lockdown meant that physical contact – touch – became something of an anathema, to be feared and avoided. Children experienced the loss of friends, extended family, structure, routine, education as well as grieving for those close to them who died or became seriously ill through infection. Furthermore, the Covid pandemic starkly exposed a range of intersectional, societal fault-lines around poverty, ethnicity, age, oppression, disability, systemic racism and social justice, the virus unforgiving in its capacity to lay bare the inequalities of our society. The full, potentially devastating mental health legacy of the pandemic in terms of child development and mental health is as yet unknown, but will no doubt become clearer over the coming years, whilst the growing need and provision of early years support is pressing.

Conversely, and from a more anecdotal perspective, I was struck by the resilience of many children, who adapted well to their new reality. I hesitantly returned to clinical practice, mindful of my own underlying health status and anxious about the new Covid safe working protocols, tooling myself up with the full range of personal protective equipment, having cleared and cleansed the therapy room and turned it into what felt like a rather unwelcoming, sterile play environment. In the waiting area, I met with my 7-year-old client, an adopted child who I have been working with long-term but had not seen for over nine months. As if it were only last week, his mother and I had to playfully search the room before I "found" him hiding behind a chair, from where he leapt out with a joyous roar. We bumped elbows and talked about the "pesky virus" that meant I had to wear a mask and which stopped us from getting too close to each other. He looked at me, shrugged and said that he was not bothered and ran out of the room and down the stairs to the playroom. "I think he is okay – I guess I had better go after him" I said to his mother.

In the playroom, he barely questioned the new layout and energetically dived into the box of play resources I had put together for him and within minutes had resumed a story we had last played nine months ago. As ever, I am continually struck by children's capacity to do what they need to do and play what they need to play. But whilst the child seamlessly picked up where we had left off, I found myself preoccupied with my own process. I felt, for want of better words, rusty and deskilled and also acutely aware of my own physicality and the awkward presence of my Parkinson's – an unwanted guest in the playroom. I felt, in the presence of this 7-year-old child, self-conscious of my bodily movement and anxious that I might be betrayed by my involuntary PD repertoire of tremors, shakes and twitches.

Play therapy, like all allied arts therapies, is an embodied process. This can be conceptualised and understood from different theoretical positions depending, perhaps, on the specific therapeutic modality. For example, within dramatherapy, Jones (1996: 152) considered the body as a "means to express, discover and develop the self . . . the body is often described as the primary means by which communication occurs between *self and other*. This is through gesture, expression and voice". Casson (2004: 166) adds that "working with the body will therefore consolidate the sense of self". Embodiment then is inexorably and intricately linked to both cognition and affect: how we think and feel about ourselves and our relationships with others, a felt sense of intra and interpersonal experience that provides a constant kinesthetic feedback loop. As Koch and Fuchs (2011) suggest, the body is the ever-constant "unifying base" of the first-person perspective that we carry with us at all times, unavoidable and inescapable – an embodied, physicalised narrative of our "self" in relation.

In contrast, Parkinson's, as a movement disorder, is all about a process of disembodiment. There is, by definition, a fundamental disconnect between neurology and physiology caused by an absence of dopamine. Simply put, there is a disruption in critical chemical messaging, which results in the body not doing what it is meant to do – faulty processing, in computer terms: Twitches, jerks, stiffness, shakes, spatial disorientation (and that is just for starters). From a personal perspective, it feels like a gradual process of disintegration of parts not working together in any kind of physically coherent, uniform way, a loss of *fluidity* one might say. That said, I am clearly much more aware of my disordered movement than are people around me, and I have little doubt that the child in the playroom noticed anything different in terms of my physical presentation. But from an embodied perspective, I was conscious as to the extent that my PD might impact upon the embodied, non-verbal process of mirrored, empathic attunement that is such an important part of the therapeutic process and this is a question that I will clearly need to explore further in relation to my potential ongoing clinical practice.

As the United Kingdom entered its second period of lockdown, my face-to-face sessions had to end and I agreed to meet with my child for fortnightly online "holding sessions"; short 20-minute sessions with the aim of maintaining some experience of therapeutic continuity until such time as we could see each other once again in person. This both confirmed and challenged my pre-held assumptions and resistance to working online. From a Parkinson's perspective, my visible symptoms were effectively, albeit temporarily, quarantined by the bordered limits of my zoom screen – my tremor virtually sanitised – although of course it was a pretence, as off-screen my symptoms persisted to a lesser or greater degree. Interestingly, when teaching and lecturing online, the tremor in my left hand and leg was always much worse than when I taught on-site, in person, which was something of a paradox. Whilst I felt much more exposed to visual scrutiny when teaching in person, there was something about the felt sense of "relational presence" that calmed me. Generally, my symptoms are exacerbated by stress and anxiety and I found the disconnected process of teaching online considerably more anxiety inducing, in the absence of any kind of relational context, and this experience seemed to support my aversion towards online working.

My client zoom sessions were a mixed experience. The child was often off-screen, accompanied by an unidentifiable range of "noises off" with the occasional socked foot hovering into view like a disembodied UFO. We played games of mime and drew pictures together, whilst siblings and parents drifted past, sometimes pausing to join in or say hello. At times my presence felt intrusive as family conflicts played out before me, sometimes drawing me in as some kind of remote therapeutic arbiter – more family therapist than play therapist. Certainly, this was not play therapy and whilst I was in some ways surprised by how well we managed to "connect", overall, my doubts around working therapeutically with children online were confirmed and highlighted issues around emotional containment, holding, confidentiality and both physical and psychological safety. But I say this, very aware that for many therapeutic disciplines and modalities, working online holds distinct advantages, possibilities and potential and in this sense Covid will clearly have a significant impact upon how the provision of therapy, in general, is conceptualised and delivered longer term. But in terms of child-centred play therapy and working individually with young children online, there are very specific theoretical, clinical and ethical challenges and it is an approach I would view with considerable caution.

## On the cold light of day

I cannot speak for other people with PD, but much of my energy during these first 18 months since my diagnosis has been mostly spent pretending not to have Parkinson's. It is exhausting. I disguise my limp, keep my left hand in my pocket a lot of the time (very noticeable in photographs), sit cross-legged to control my shaking leg, try not to fall over when putting my socks on, and so it goes. My daily life has become a series of strategic "work-arounds", partly as a way of coping and partly to convey a sense of "normality", although who I am trying to convince, I am not quite sure. I guess it is all part of the process: denial, anger, bargaining, depression, acceptance etc. Is that the order they are meant to be in? Is it that neat? I seem to be trapped in a continuous cycle of denial, depression and acceptance – and repeat. I am not sure where the anger has gone, which is probably a worry. And who am I supposed to bargain with? Myself? How does that work? The problem being that, unlike a single event, Parkinson's is progressive, incremental – steps, strides, jumps, leaps and the occasional plateau (they are nice), but all in the same inevitable direction. Suddenly I find myself typing with one finger, or I go swimming and realise that I cannot swim backstroke anymore, my arms and legs simply unable to work together in unison. Simple acts of coordination seem to have suddenly become things I need to think consciously about as if the disease is goading me with its own very special brand of mundane torture. Maybe, like Dennis Potter's cancer, I should give it a name and externalise it. Potter famously named his tumour "Rupert", after Rupert Murdoch, for whom he held a strong dislike (understandably, some might think). What should I call my Parkinson's? Donald? Boris? Piers? No, perhaps that is a step too far.

But as I say, hiding the symptoms, either from myself or those around me, is hard work and as we move out of the cover of lockdown into the cold light of day, I find myself having to struggle again with the visible realities of my condition. This is compounded by a degree of social anxiety, having had very limited offline contact with other people for the last year, and I feel dazzled by the intense glare of the outside world. As I return to my lecturing role, navigating around the university's complex one-way system, I find myself having to negotiate much more than just corridors, stairs and no-entry signs. Indeed, it is a whole new emotional and psychological landscape and I feel acutely physically self-conscious, deskilled and anxious as I have to reengage with the outside world. The eerie quiet and empty spaces of the university bring to mind images of the Mary Celeste, adrift and deserted, and when I finally negotiate the snakes and ladders signage and reach my office, my cluttered desk sits untouched after nearly a year, like some kind of time capsule from another, less cluttered age.

Emerging out of lockdown, I am also confronted with new questions around the experience of illness and how open I should be with colleagues, students and clients. I have had to think carefully about self-disclosure and about issues of power and vulnerability in the face of my own felt sense of fallibility. Certainly, I am not the omnipotent therapist, and have never claimed to be (who would?) but I have had cause to consider carefully the impact of my illness on both clients and trainees and how this might be experienced. It is all very well being the "wounded healer" (Jung, 1951), but what, I wonder, might it be like for clients to perceive me as the 'wounded therapist'?

As Wilton writes about her own experience of illness:

I think the fact of my evidently not being the healthy, invulnerable strong one as was put upon me sometimes before I became ill helped to equalise the power balance between my patient and myself in some cases and at times, I used my vulnerability to bring this about. What I am saying is that my sensed powerlessness as a result of illness enabled the other in some cases to more easily have his or her power.

(2001: 1)

So perhaps there will be some inevitable shifts in the balance of the therapeutic relationship, indeed in all my relationships, and a sense of recalibration as I seek to find a way of being alongside my illness . . . and perhaps, within my client work, potential opportunities for conversations about vulnerability, fragility, fear and hope.

Clinical supervision has been helpful in this regard; being able to express my feelings of vulnerability and self-doubt and to voice my concerns about fitness to practice as a therapist. Being something of an introvert by nature, I can all too easily lose a sense of external perspective and objectivity and become overwhelmed by my tendency to catastrophise and see only the worst possible outcomes (I am also easily prone to pessimism). Conversations with my supervisor have helped to normalise a far from normal situation and provide a grounded sense of what is possible, manageable and appropriate, in terms of both my own process and that of my clients. Being able to look ahead and think about what I need to be able to practice safely and effectively has been invaluable, whether this be in terms of physical support and adjustments, emotional support or managing my caseload. But critically, these conversations have given me a sense of hope, possibility and confidence in my future work as a therapist and have helped me to believe that my diagnosis does not have to be the terminal, career-ending bullet that I initially felt it to be.

I have little doubt that many therapists are having (or have had) to face the challenge of personal illness, in all its many forms, and it is an experience that tests our resilience to its very limits. It is important then that we gain strength from where we can. Elsewhere in this book, colleagues have written about personal experiences of vulnerability, shame and self-care, amongst others, and when as therapists we are hit by life-changing events that knock us of course, or pull us out of shape, it is important that we are able to seek support, in whatever form that might take, to navigate our way forward.

## Final thoughts

Throughout all this, having to co-edit a book on personal process might seem timely, but in other ways it has felt an almost impossible, absurdly paradoxical task, within the ever-changing, shifting landscape that we have all had to negotiate over recent times. I and my editorial colleague and indeed all the contributors to this book have (like everyone) felt overwhelmed by personal process over the course of the pandemic, and this chapter is just one story of many. Personally, it has been hard to create the space, time and emotional distance to reflect on the ever-moving reality of both my own situation and the wider, national and international picture, and my central challenge within this chapter has been around personal proximity to the writing and how I position myself within the words, which once said, cannot be taken back. As I said in my introduction, I wondered if writing this might be a part of my "coming out" – the beginnings of acceptance – but in truth I am still not sure how helpful it has been. Time will tell. Certainly, it has been challenging, forcing me to hold my gaze with the unknowable and the intolerable, like a childhood staring contest to see who will blink or look away first. But of course, Parkinson's will never blink or look away, so it is not a game that I am ever going to win, and that in itself is about acceptance. I am also aware that I have taken what feels like a considerable risk with this chapter, in terms of self-disclosure but that, in essence, is what this book is about – the personal process of the therapist – and all that this means.

*Postscript*

*Earlier in this chapter I made reference to a planned 70-mile hike across the Lake District along the Cumbria Way – as I said, more in hope than expectation. But I am pleased to report that I successfully completed the hike, in the company of good friends. There is a truth to be found in walking, and perhaps the truth I discovered is that there is life beyond my diagnosis; that it does not have to define who I am and what I can be. Julian Barnes may have well written "what happiness is there in just the memory of happiness?". Well, I guess I just have to keep creating new memories.*

## References

Barnes, J. (2014) *Levels of Life*. New York: Vintage.

Benjamin, J. (2017) *Beyond Doer and Done To: Recognition Theory, Intersubjectivity and the Third*. London: Routledge.

Casson, J. (2004) *Drama, Psychotherapy and Psychosis*. Hove: Brunner-Routledge.

Guggenbuhl-Craig, A. (1979) *Power in the Helping Professions*. Irving, TX: Spring (first published 1971).

Jones, P. (1996) *Drama as Therapy: Theatre as Living*. London: Routledge.

Jung, C. (1951) *Fundamental Questions of Psychotherapy*. Princeton, NJ: Princeton University Press.

Koch, S. C. & Fuchs, T. (2011) Embodied Arts Therapies. *The Arts in Psychotherapy*, 38, pp. 276–280.

Maslow, A. H. (1962) *Toward a Psychology of Being*. Princeton: D. Van Nostrand Company.

Rajkumar, R. P. (2020) Attachment Theory and Psychological Responses to the COVID-19 Pandemic: A Narrative Review. *Psychiatria Danubina*, 32(2), pp. 256–261.

Wilton, A. (2001) The Impact of Illness on the Therapist's Self and the Handling and Use of This in Therapy. *Reformulation, ACAT News*, Autumn, p. x.

Woskett, V. (1999) *The Therapeutic Use of Self: Counselling Practice, Research and Supervision*. London: Routledge.

# Chapter 12

# When we say goodbye

## A reflective account of endings in the therapeutic relationship

*Martine Wheeldon*

## Introduction

*This chapter shares some accounts of the writer's personal experiences in practice and interpretations from research. All client and participant details have been anonymised and altered to remove any identifying information.*

As I sit and mull over how I might start a chapter on endings, that will ultimately lead to the end of this book, I find myself reflecting on how my perception of endings in the therapeutic process has changed in so many ways and wonder if I will still be able to relate to the words of my trainee play therapist self. Much has changed in my world, professionally and personally since I completed my play therapy training in 2018, most significantly that I have become a mother. Throughout this chapter I will give accounts of endings in my practice pre-parenthood, during pregnancy and as a parent. I understand that for some readers, my accounts and experiences may trigger emotional responses connected to their own experiences in this area. I will try hard to recall and be sensitive to the feelings evoked for me when working with, and particularly saying goodbye to children, when I did not have my own.

Throughout this chapter I will not only draw on my own experiences of endings in practice but also utilise the more generalised findings from my research project, undertaken whilst studying a masters in play therapy at the University of Roehampton. I chose to focus on the topic of endings for my research project as I had been impacted so greatly by the endings that I had experienced with my clients in my first practice placement and felt I needed to further understand what this was about. I found that endings were the part of my practice that I found most difficult. I remember feeling particularly rejected and persecuted when one of my clients wished to end prematurely, and a sense of failure and desire to continue with another client, who had not made the progress I had hoped for in the 12-week time frame we had.

I wondered if I was alone in these feelings of self-doubt and thoughts of "what if" or "have I done enough". I had read about the "good enough ending" (Lanyado, 2004) and could rationalise that there was no such thing as the perfect ending, but wondered how other play therapists made peace with those endings that

DOI: 10.4324/9781003017271-12

did not feel entirely positive. Was this something that developed over time, with confidence built over years of post-qualification experience, or was it something specific to me. Would I ever feel as though the experience of ending with a child that I had built a meaningful relationship with was a positive one?

Prior to beginning my training, I had been undergoing fertility treatment, which had been unsuccessful. I had not given up on my desire to become a mother but had postponed treatment to pursue my other desire, to become a play therapist. I had worked with children who had experienced trauma and attachment difficulties in an educational provision for many years and had never experienced my personal circumstances impacting on my role, so did not expect it to in this situation either. However, I quickly realised that due to the nature of the interactions conducive to the therapeutic relationship, I would have to acknowledge my own desire for that connection with another and be conscious of it throughout my work with a child, and particularly the ending process.

Throughout this chapter I will share the key themes that emerged from my research and discuss how these themes relate or have related in the past, to my own experiences of ending with a client in play therapy. I will also touch on how becoming pregnant post-qualification and preparing for endings with clients because of my impending maternity leave, triggered very different feelings within me.

## Theoretical underpinnings

With little written about how play therapists might feel about endings, I was left reading articles about "therapeutic change" and "positive termination" and feeling as if I needed to do a lot more work in my personal therapy and that I was not cut out for the emotional impact that play therapy entailed. I also wondered if I was a poor therapist, not capable of achieving these positive endings that were spoken of frequently in the literature. This led me to want to know more about how qualified play therapists experienced endings with their clients, once the pressure in training to meet a certain amount of placement hours is lifted, as well as if other personal experiences may have impacted on the play therapists' ability to end with their clients.

Endings in therapy have provoked meaningful discussion in psychoanalytic, arts therapies and recently play therapy texts, with many considering how a "good enough" (Lanyado, 2004: 126) ending can occur. Some key contributors to play therapy texts (West, 1996; Landreth, 2002; Oaklander, 2007) have discussed the difficulties that endings can evoke for children, with many contributing practical advice to help play therapists support their clients through this process.

The impact that the relationship between play therapist and client can have has also been discussed in many texts, with the therapeutic relationship often likened to the attachment relationship formed between the infant and the caregiver (Mallinckrodt et al., 1995). Attachment theory developed by Bowlby (1969, 1988) and Ainsworth (1979) highlights the need for secure, predictable and attuned care, providing the child with the "secure base" (Bowlby, 1988) needed to go on and explore the world with confidence.

The caring, accepting and supportive (Axline, 1989; Landreth, 2002) qualities of the play therapist, that enable connections (O'Connor & Schaefer, 1994) to form between the client and the therapist, can equally provide the secure base needed for children to successfully end play therapy feeling more confident and prepared for their future. However, the sense of loss that client and therapist may feel when play therapy comes to an end is acknowledged (West, 1996; Oaklander, 2007; Landreth, 2002), and discussions regarding how to sensitively prepare clients for the separation or "bridging stage" (West, 1996: 111) can be found in many play therapy texts.

I wondered though, how the play therapist might expect to prepare for the ending of a caring and attuned relationship with a child client, likened to that of a parent-child relationship; particularly if this was the first time the therapist had experienced a relationship of this kind. To prepare myself for the feelings that I might encounter, I looked to existing play therapy texts, hoping that I might find advice, or at least other accounts of the way endings had impacted play therapists, but found little. With the emphasis in texts being around the child feeling supported and in control of the final sessions (Landreth, 2002; Oaklander, 2007) a consideration that is extremely valid, it appears that there is less reflection of the therapists' experiences of ending. Some thoughtful contributions and research have been conducted in adult and broader child psychotherapy disciplines (Cangelsoi, 1997; Bamford & Akhurst, 2014); however, it is sparse and either not current or specific to play therapy.

The aim of my research therefore was to explore how practicing play therapists approached endings with their clients and for me to develop a greater understanding of what play therapists believe are the most important considerations for them when ending with a client, as well as what emotional responses may be evoked for them as they say goodbye to clients with whom they have formed a therapeutic relationship.

I anticipated that key themes such as loss and anxiety might be triggered in play therapists who had developed attachment like relationships, as discussed similarly by Marmarosh (2017) or feelings of "severed relationship[s] . . . vulnerability [and] self-doubt" as found in Bamford and Akhurst's study of school-based counsellors (2014: 465). However, I do not think I fully appreciated how beneficial Interpretative Phenomenological Analysis (IPA) research methodology would be, in evoking and enabling detailed accounts of personal experience, until I began interviewing participants. As Smith and Eatough (2007) discussed, IPA research often requires the participant to take a role in the interpretation of their own phenomenology, and the researcher then focuses on each individual case and how the participant makes sense of their personal and social world (Smith & Eatough, 2007) before attempting to find similarities or differences with other cases (Wheeldon, 2018).

As I move into the main section of this chapter, I shall attempt to weave in the key themes that emerged from my research and how they relate to personal accounts of my own clinical experience.

## What are the most important considerations for play therapists as they end with their clients?

In answer to this first question, four predominate themes emerged from my research.

### *Preparation*

Preparation for the ending was discussed as an important factor. Most participants felt that pre-set time frames were containing for both them and the child, as they knew how much time they had and could prepare effectively for the ending. Ray states that the "goal of therapy is to end therapy" (2014: 230) and therefore it is useful to have the ending in the child's and therapist's sights from the beginning. Clausen et al. (2012) speak, however, of certain groups of clients, such as children in care or with multiple layers of trauma or loss, where short-term interventions would not be appropriate. I now see, after working post-qualification, the value of having these experiences, to prepare a trainee play therapist for working under financial or resource constraints that may come with working within a clinic or mental health context. However, during training I believe that the lack of flexibility I felt in this area prevented me from seeing the value of containment that time frames can provide.

The feelings that I earlier referred to – of feeling rejected and persecuted when one of my client's wished to end prematurely, and a sense of failure and desire to continue with another client, who had not made the progress I had hoped for in the short time we had available – were triggered by having a set time frame of placement hours, which with one client I was unable to meet and for another did not seem enough. As an inexperienced trainee, it felt unnerving for me that my placement hours and experiences were not going to fit neatly into the metaphorical boxes I had allocated for them. I felt that by not meeting my placement hours as set out and expected by the university, therapy had "failed" in some way. I remember wondering if, for my first client, sessions were becoming too painful for her and as an inexperienced play therapist, I was not equipped to manage these feelings sensitively enough to encourage her to continue. As West suggests, the "inadequate play therapist", lacking skill and unable to serve the client's best interests (1996: 20). As I lacked confidence, this feeling of failing my client in some way felt very real.

As I look back, I can see my former self donning my imaginary superhero cape ready to save the world. I naively thought that it would be solely me helping the young clients I worked with and forgot, at times, the importance of truly keeping the ethos of client-centred therapy at the heart of my work. I felt under pressure, both internally and externally, to build a meaningful relationship with the child I was working with, a relationship that would feel positive and help the child grow, and on occasion forgot that the real change comes from within the young person. It was through experience and further understanding that I was able to accept that change very rarely fits into pre-determined time frames; sometimes change is noticed sooner and often much later than expected, and therefore having flexibility around the ending process is extremely valuable.

I was unable to fully accept this until the pressures of training were lifted and I no longer felt the great sense of responsibility to prove that I was a good play therapist to meet my own needs. I felt more at ease in the metaphorical dance that the therapeutic relationship requires, being able to follow the client's lead and move in and out of responding in certain ways; much like the attuned parent-child relationship, but without feeling the need for the relationship to be a certain way or lead to any one thing. As one participant in my research discussed, "natural endings" that have not been pre-set, often come when the therapist, along with client and parents, begin noticing change.

### Noticing change

Noticing change as an indicator of success was another factor that participants placed importance on – "if I have built something really positive, it feels okay to let them go". Many methods of tracking change are available to play therapists (Nordling & Guerney, 1999; Dighton, 2001; Cochran et al., 2010) and it is thought useful to track change to demonstrate the effectiveness of the treatment method. Within my research, participants spoke of feeling that the change noticed was sometimes too small to be reflected on a change tracking form, but that noticing it still helped.

When undertaking research into the "drop-out rates" of children in therapy, Campbell et al. (2000) found that determining change is complicated and that play therapists may class endings as premature when they have not noticed change. However, the parent or child may have noticed or felt change, suggesting that the therapist's inability to see change could be more to do with the therapist's "reluctance to close or end the relationship" (Campbell et al., 2000: 135).

Upon reflection, the first ever client I worked with made huge strides towards positive change during the time I spent with her. At the time though, I missed many of the subtle signs indicating that the once sad, lonely, young person was quickly starting to feel more confident, make friends and subsequently want to be with them rather than in therapy with me. This was a positive ending for her; she was ready, able to develop friendships and rely on a wider circle of support rather than an hour a week therapy session.

For me it was an earlier than planned ending, which firstly meant that I did not complete my placement hours and secondly left me feeling rejected; was I not a good enough therapist for her to want to continue seeing me? Would a different play therapist have been able to build a stronger more effective relationship that kept her in therapy for the allocated 12 sessions at least?

Through weekly supervision and personal therapy, I began to work through my feelings related to this ending and gained a greater awareness of my personal desire for the young people that I worked with to form attachments with me, as this was something I felt I was missing. Once again, it might be suggested that I was losing sight of the child as the focus of the work. However, through noticing the juxtaposition of the client's and their family's observations of change, compared to my own feelings of despair, I was able to gain a better understanding of what was triggered for me from my own experiences. This enabled me to be mindful of my own responses when starting to explore the ending process and how they might like it be. This client expressed their desire to sit in on the final review session with their parents and hear all the positive feedback and changes that had been noticed. This, for a child who had potentially felt unnoticed for some time, due to the emotional needs of parents and then, although not voiced, by me as well, was an important opportunity to feel, seen and heard.

### Client's control and choice

Participants spoke of how facilitating opportunities for their clients to have control over the ending was important – "the best endings are when they decide for themselves" (Wheeldon, 2018: 25). The importance of giving choice and promoting a child's autonomy during the ending phase has been discussed by others (West, 1996; Landreth, 2002), with Landreth stating that the "termination" phase should follow a child-centred approach and that the ending should be as unique to the child as the relationship has been (West, 1996).

The research found that play therapists feel better about the ending when clients can make choices about when or how the ending takes place, even on occasions where endings feel premature. Ray (2014) discusses different types of "premature endings" and suggests that "forced endings", due to external factors such as funding cuts or venue disruption, or endings initiated by the therapist because of changes in their own circumstances, lead to greater feelings of "rejection" and "guilt" (Ray, 2014: 236).

In the three years since conducting my research and working with young people who have predominately experienced developmental trauma and attachment difficulties, I have found that as every child is unique, every ending with them is also unique. The way one child copes with and wants the ending to be can be very different from another, and at times this is surprising to the therapist.

When I first met a young man, whom I shall call Billy, I knew that the work was likely to be long term. He had experienced significant abuse, neglect and loss, and consequently found it very hard to trust most adults and would seek opportunities to control and orchestrate situations to push them away; all except his father with whom Billy was desperate for love and approval, despite his father's constant rejections and violent behaviours. For the first four sessions Billy refused any eye contact, self-soothed by picking at his nails profusely and dismissed most of my verbal reflections, telling me that I was wrong and did not know anything. He would also at times make loud scoffing noises preventing me from sharing my reflections. I often felt as though I was worthless and getting it wrong, experiencing the transference of Billy's own feelings towards his father. However, Billy continued to return each week and began to take control of the process by initiating time at the beginning of the sessions where he would explore the sensory materials. Billy stated that I was not to speak; otherwise I would see how angry he could become, and if I remained silent, then he would share the sensory materials with me. This communicated an experience and relationship that in some ways resembled the domestic abuse that Billy had witnessed in early life, as well as communicating his own feelings of oppression and ambivalence in his father's presence. As much as I wanted to challenge Billy's dictating behaviour, I also always wanted to form a connection with him, as I imagine he felt towards his father.

After working with Billy for four weeks, I discovered I was pregnant. I spoke to my supervisor and manager who both encouraged me to think carefully about the value of continuing work at this time, alongside the potential risks. However, I felt a great desire to continue working with Billy, as he returned to our sessions each week and whilst reluctant, appeared to be developing trust, as he demonstrated to me his feelings of frustration verbally and through his use of sensory materials. I felt I had to give Billy the opportunity to work through whatever it was that was drawing him to attend each week and to provide him with an autonomous experience that was not derived from power struggles, but within a relationship in which the adult wanted him to succeed. I knew that the relationship would come to an end in around 30 weeks but hoped that through preparation and understanding this could be different to the rushed, premature endings and loss that we had both previously experienced.

I was shocked when Billy's response to me telling him I was pregnant was that he already knew. He did not wish to speak any more about it or ask any questions and continued to re-engage in working through the sensory materials as he did at the beginning of each session. The following week however, Billy came to me and announced that he had been doing his research and estimated that our time would come to an end on a date not too far from the date I had planned to end direct work, a date I had not shared with him. We talked together about how a little bit of time is needed to prepare for a baby's arrival and Billy spoke about his own experiences of younger siblings being born as he utilised the toy dolls in the playroom, comparing them to his siblings as babies. Whilst Billy played with the dolls, he was tentative, speaking of the facts that his mother had shared with him about pregnancy and childbirth and of his own wish to be a father someday. Billy did not present in an overly dictating way but seemed more excited to be able to share something with me that he appeared confident in the knowledge of. He took control of the ending by establishing a date that felt comfortable for him and that he could prepare for and in this sense, Billy was also able to exert his autonomy over the process and find a way for us to maintain our relationship. It surprised me however that my pregnancy never appeared to cause conflict in our work despite Billy not being able to reside with his mother unlike his younger siblings. This demonstrated the loyalty that Billy felt towards his father, as well as his possible fantasies about becoming a father himself and seeing my pregnancy as more of a parallel to his own desires of becoming a parent, rather than a maternal rejection.

Whilst at the time this ending felt positive, in so far as the client was in control, there were multiple layers of intersubjectivity and self-disclosure within the relationship that came from the client's awareness of the impending reason for the work to cease. There were also other losses and endings that were experienced by the client external to therapy, but none were explored in the same way as they might have been, if the work was not time restricted or could have been left open. Billy was given the opportunity to continue working with a colleague of mine but chose to maintain his decision to end therapy on the allocated date he had decided on.

## Parents

Within my research, the impact of parents or carers on the therapeutic process and particularly ending was mentioned. Participants spoke of how feeling that the parents or carers of a client being on board and supportive of the work, as well as them noticing change, often helped endings feel more positive and prompted the therapist's decision to start preparing a client and their parents for this process. Just as the need for parental commitment is part of the play therapy assessment, the effectiveness of a "positive parental alliance" has been discussed by Myrick (2017) as well as Sloves and Bellinger Peterlin (1994), when exploring parent work with adolescents in psychotherapy and the importance placed on the parent's willingness to engage.

My longest case during training was with a client that I shall name Sam. Sam embraced everything about his time in play therapy; he was small for his age and had an abundance of energy that he used to play with everything in the playroom. Sam initially pulled on my maternal urge to protect him, due to his vulnerable presentation and uncertainty, often checking out what he hoped to play with me before doing so. Sam made great changes over his time in therapy; he developed an increasing autonomy and some of his fears and anxieties reduced. Sam was supported phenomenally by his teacher and most importantly his mother, clearly two very strong, significant female figures in his life.

Throughout my work with Sam, over a period of 35 weeks, I also built good relationships with both these important people in his life. Sam's teacher was observant and sensitive to his responses before and after his play therapy sessions and would send me regular reports to let me know how he was getting on or any changes that she noticed in the classroom. Sam's mother grew in confidence each time I met with her and always embraced the playful nature of the work in her responses to Sam and with myself in review meetings. Due to all parties' commitment, I felt able to plan and prepare for the ending in advance with all of them.

In his sessions, Sam used containers and marbles to signify each session that had gone by, placing a marble for each session into a container so that he had a visual representation of how many sessions he had left. As we approached the ending, Sam asked if his mother would be able to join him for his final play therapy session. I wondered aloud about what it was that Sam would gain from having his mother in his final session, and he said that he wanted me to help teach her some of the games that we had played together. Sam's mother had been forthcoming in her involvement in review meetings and trying things at home with Sam and it may be that he had noticed the changes in his mother, in a similar way that we had noticed positive changes in him. Landreth shares his thoughts on parental involvement in therapy stating that "when parents feel better about themselves, are less anxious, and are better adjusted, they are more likely to respond in positive, self-enhancing ways to their children" (2002: 154). It was as though we were celebrating both of their newfound sense of selves and enlightened way of being together. Sam also expressed his delight when he realised that by his mother joining us, he would be the first of his siblings to be collected that day, as she usually collected his youngest sibling first. This gave an opportunity for both Sam and his mother to share some unique uninterrupted time together within the playroom, as they both stepped away from the therapeutic process.

As I approached the ending session with Sam, I felt a great deal of apprehension about how I might manage my own emotions when saying goodbye to this little boy, towards whom I experienced genuine feelings of maternal care, and to some degree towards his mother also. Also, however, Sam's request gave me a different focus, a way to hand back those maternal feelings I might have felt for Sam to his mother and support her to carry on some of the work with Sam that I had started. West (1996) talks about the bridging phase of the process, as the therapist and child move out of the therapy room together. But in this instance, Sam's mother moved into the therapy room to support him to move out of it.

## What feelings emerge for play therapists as they end work with a child?

Considering the previous attachment-related research (Mallinckrodt et al., 1995) in play therapy and studies related to adult psychotherapy (Marmarosh, 2017), it is not surprising that when participants reflected on endings with children with whom they had formed attachments, ambivalent feelings occurred.

Oaklander (2007) discusses how inexperienced play therapists may feel the need to supress their own feelings about the ending, to prevent the child feeling guilty or worried. She argues however that by play therapists not being in touch with and addressing their own feelings in relation to the ending can make "termination more difficult" (Oaklander, 2007: 204).

### Responsibility

Participants shared a sense of responsibility to ensure that positive changes occurred within, and external to, the playroom. Whilst issues of responsibility do not seem to have been found in other studies, Bamford and Akhurst (2014) did find that school-based counsellors also had similar responses of "parental feelings of concern", considering the "depth of the relationship" with the children they worked with. Cangelsoi (1997) discusses the personal feelings that child psychotherapists may have when saying goodbye to a child, with whom they have developed a personal connection and likens this to the struggle that parents often have in "letting go" of their children (Cangelsoi, 1997: 31) at key developmental stages.

Participants spoke of it feeling easier to let go of clients and felt a sense of relief when they knew that there were strong attachments within the client's own families, and people willing to support them, as was my experience with Sam and his mother. Ray writes of how when a play therapist feels that they provide the only predictability and stability in a child's life, it can be difficult to want to end with the client, stating that "there is a tendency for some therapists to prolong therapy until the child's situation is perfect" (Ray, 2014: 237).

I remember feeling after my first year in training that having experienced two endings that challenged me to be flexible, reflective and from my perspective, fight for a good enough ending, that I would now be prepared to manage any kind of ending thrown at me. However, whilst the endings may not have met my expectations, there were other people around the child who could hold and support them, whether that be their parents or other safe adults such as a teacher or clinical professional.

In my second placement, I experienced strong feelings of parental concern and protection, towards a child I was working with, whom I shall call Betsy. I felt an attachment forming that I had not experienced with any other client. Betsy attended every one of her sessions, initially looking to me for guidance and reassurance, and over time developing confidence in her own autonomy and utilising play to explore and make sense of her world, inviting me to play alongside her. I felt utterly devastated when I was informed that her challenging behaviours in the classroom deemed her unsafe to remain in school and therefore could no longer attend our play therapy sessions. I fought what felt like a monumental battle to help the headteacher understand the importance of Betsy being able to attend an ending session and ensured that the ending was as positive as possible for this little girl who was being pulled away from me before we reached that "perfect" ending that I longed for, and that perhaps she did too.

For Betsy, I held a tea party and brought along cake and apple juice as she had requested. She took time to play with everything that she had played with in her sessions prior, one last time before sitting down for her party. She took her time with every piece of food and shared it out with me precisely. In that last session, I felt as though time stood still and we were given the time to really connect with another, even though we both knew that we would be saying goodbye. For all my clients, I provide a box at the beginning of our time together which they can decorate and personalise, and this then becomes the place where any of their creations within the therapy room are kept. I suggested that Betsy look through her box and decide if there was anything that she would like to keep before the end. She meticulously went through every painting, drawing and model and shared her memories of them before deciding what she might like to keep and what she would leave with me for safe keeping. I knew a long time before that moment that I would never forget Betsy, but in our time together in our final session, Betsy showed me that she would remember our time together too, that despite our relationship ending before I feel either of us were ready, it was an important relationship for us both. We had both learned and developed in each other's presence, and Betsy ensured that we would both have reminders of our time together.

## Wanting to remember

Participants placed importance on helping clients remember their play therapy within the final ending session and beyond, as well as being able to remember the clients themselves, "holding" clients in mind, and "taking something from them". West (1996) writes of the use of tangible reminders, which relates to the participants in this study who spoke of either giving a card or encouraging the client to leave a symbol of themselves behind, in order that both could remember the experience and relationship.

Norcross et al. (2017) found that more encouragement needs to be placed on trainee therapists to enable them to verbally explore the journey that they had taken with their clients in the ending phase of treatment. Yet for the play therapists in this study, and in keeping with play being the language of children (Landreth, 2002), examples of more creative means were given when sharing feelings and experiences with child clients.

As part of my practice, I like to share an ending letter with my client in our final session together, inspired by Oaklander (2007), and will include images, perhaps hand drawn, a copy of something taken from the child's sessions or a published image of a particular character if the child has shown specific interest. The purpose of the ending letter is for me to demonstrate what I have learnt about the child, what I will remember of them and to share the progress or changes that I notice. The only time I have been unable to do this, which is with great regret, is when working with a client whilst pregnant in my first post-qualification role. I will name this client Jo. Jo was aware that I would be leaving the organisation for a period whilst on maternity leave. Whilst I had spoken to her about the ending process and my uncertainty of when I might return, Jo refused to say goodbye stating that she wanted to continue to work with me upon my return. Seven months into my maternity leave, the world was faced with the COVID-19 pandemic and the country went into a state of lockdown. I was therefore unable to return to work as planned and visit Jo as promised. I had also decided that I would not be returning to my previous role due to travel and childcare difficulties. I tried to contact Jo, but she did not wish to speak over the telephone, perhaps feeling let down or rejected by me, so sent my ending letter, but have no knowledge of how this was received. This made me feel a great sense of guilt and disappointment in myself that I had been unable to keep the pathway to work open as I had promised and did not know what happened next to Jo or how she felt about the ending.

## Shifts in perspective post-qualification

The biggest shift that I have experienced, probably unsurprisingly, is how my initial drive for maternal connection has reduced. Because I have become a mother, it does not mean however that my hopes for building meaningful relationships with young people that emulate the care and nurture provided by a positive attachment relationship have gone. I am just perhaps more aware of the need for balance, ensuring emotional boundaries for myself as much as the client. I have learnt about the importance of ensuring that the child in therapy has an adult outside of the playroom who is able to hold and support them emotionally in some way and acknowledge now that as much as the therapeutic relationship resembles the attachment relationship in that hour, the benefits for the child to have an adult that provides this consistently is what is most important. This leads me to hold less responsibility for the child in therapy and in turn I feel prepared to hand more of that responsibility back to the parent or carer as the ending approaches.

In the four years I have been practicing play therapy, whilst training and post-qualification, I feel lucky to be able to say that I have enjoyed my work with each of my clients and experienced genuine care and joy in their company. I cannot say however that I am sure the children that I have worked would always say the same and know that sometimes endings may bring a great sense of relief for the play therapist or the child. But that does not mean that the work has not been beneficial, just that the relationship may have evoked something different for them. I have experienced endings that have been planned, due to the wishes of the child and my own personal circumstances, and endings that have not been so planned and I have had to find flexible, creative ways of ensuring an ending in some way. In every ending I have felt sadness to be saying goodbye to a child that I have cared for, however external and internal factors have impacted on the depth of that sadness and how much pleasure the ending might have also brought to myself, the child and their family, by noticing positive changes and growth.

I have experienced three stages of life whilst practicing play therapy and subsequently three different ways of experiencing endings. The first stage being pre-qualification when I was impacted by feelings of failure when endings occurred, particularly in the shorter cases where a child chose to end early, or time ran out before change could occur. I believe that, despite my lack of experience, all endings at this time of my life would have been a challenge for me, as they reminded me of the maternal connection that I longed for. This is my personal experience and potentially over time with the support of supervision, personal therapy and developing confidence in my ability I may have been able to overcome or put these feelings to one side, as I am sure many other therapists are able to do. Nevertheless, I feel that it is important to highlight the need for congruence on the therapist's part when considering endings, as had I not been able to explore the way in which endings were triggering these, sometimes debilitating, feelings of unworthiness in me I may have continued to experience similar feelings in my practice leading to my belief that I was not a worthwhile therapist.

The second stage is when I was practicing during pregnancy and whilst I still had difficult feelings towards the endings, they were ambivalent as I knew that I was ending the sessions and leaving the organisation to be able to experience great joy and attachment for myself. I felt guilt for leaving children that I knew did not have similar attachments and at times wished that the reason for us ending work could be different, to reduce the anguish and guilt I felt at choosing my own children over them. This is when I was able to reflect on those positive endings when the child felt held by another, as I was able to relinquish some of my feelings of responsibility knowing that thankfully, in many cases, the child will have other adults in their life who care for them. The therapeutic relationship and the interactions that occur within the therapeutic hour may evoke similar feelings for both the therapist and the child, of a caring and attuned attachment relationship; yet the goal with any attachment relationship is for the caregiver to provide the child with the confidence and a sense of security to move on to explore the world and their surroundings independently. The "good enough ending" for me now is not so much about the strength of the therapeutic relationship, but about whether the client has developed in areas that will allow them to navigate and cope better in the wider world.

The third stage, as a mother, comes with a greater understanding of the importance of the parent-child attachment and that whilst the therapeutic relationship may mirror this in some way, it is more beneficial if a child is able to receive this relationship from their care giver. This stage is still relatively new to me, and I constantly question whether I am a "good enough" parent in my personal world, let alone in my professional one. Becoming a parent has raised a whole new array of insecurities and has perhaps allowed me to be more sensitive, and reflective of the needs of the parents or carers in my client's lives. I now incorporate Developmental Dyadic Psychotherapy (DDP) (Dan Hughes, 2006) into my work with parents and carers, which I find helpful in being able to facilitate some distance in my work with the child. I work with parents or carers to equip them with the skills to build and develop consistent attachment relationships, knowing now that whilst the loving care and attention that the child experiences during their play therapy is extremely valuable, it is equally important, if not more so, for them to experience this in their day-to-day life.

## Conclusion

When I initially embarked on the journey to write a chapter on endings, reflecting on my experiences over three years of practice, I believed that I would mainly conclude that reduced pressures and a greater confidence would be the most prevalent aspects of my discussion. Over time and the opportunity to explore my own personal process, I must acknowledge that for me the biggest impact has not been whether I had an academic deadline looming over my head, but more personal deadlines and ones related to my trajectory to parenthood that took precedence.

I accept that my own experiences and feelings are personal to me and may not resonate in the same way for others. Still, through my research and conversations with other play therapists, I believe that many of the readers of this book will have been encouraged to become play therapists because of their innate desires to be in the presence of children. Desires to share moments of varying emotion, to support and care for the child in their presence in ways that help them to grow, develop and achieve their self-actualising tendencies. If the most valuable thing about play therapy is the therapeutic relationship between child and therapist, which many believe is so, then of course whatever the play therapist as well as the child brings into the playroom will impact on the relationship. Play therapists, therefore, need to be mindful of their own process and what they bring to the ending with their client, in relation to their own experiences.

As I found through my research, the desire to create an ending for clients that feels "good enough", giving the client choice and control over the process and finding ways to form links to the relationship and the work that takes place in the playroom, feels very important. The way play therapists approach endings practically may vary, with some wishing to provide physical, tangible remind-ers for the child, through letters or gifts, and others hoping to bridge the child's transition from the playroom to their outside world, through stepping out with the child in varying ways, or in my case allowing a parent in. Many play therapists not only witness and acknowledge the difficult feelings that endings might evoke in children but also, myself included, strive to find ways to share with the child the success of the work, by identifying changes and highlighting the journey they have been on.

My research provided me with a unique opportunity to gain insight into the feelings and experiences of other play therapists. However, there were still ten-dencies to move the focus back to the client's experience of the ending, which raised questions about whether this is an inherent quality of the child-centred play therapists – to "constantly consider the needs and feeling of their clients before their own; or might difficulties around articulating their own feelings regarding the loss of the relationship relate to the difficult, ambivalent feelings that endings can create?" (Wheeldon, 2018: 52). Through exploring my own experiences and feelings related to endings, I have certainly felt an element of shame at times, allowing myself to be preoccupied by my own process rather than that of the child's. However, it is through exploring my personal processes in retrospect and particularly at the time that enabled me to make decisions based on mine and the child's best interests. Some of my ending experiences with clients felt too soon, some did not feel good enough, some put the child's needs and wishes at the heart of the process, and some came because of my personal need to end. Each ending was unique to the relationship I had with that child and no ending has ever looked the same. Because of that I acknowledge that endings are, and probably always will be, an ever-evolving part of my process and practice.

I am unsure if I will ever feel as though an ending is truly "good enough", but as long as I am able to provide children with a space in which they feel cared for, supported and free to explore their experiences and emotions through play, the ending will also come. But I take solace in this closing statement from one research participant.

*'[T]o end is better than not to start, you know'*

(Wheeldon, 2018: 54)

## References

Ainsworth, M. D. S. (1979) Infant – Mother Attachment. *American Psychologist*, 34(10), pp. 932–937. Available at: www.psy.miami.edu/faculty/dmessinger/c_c/rsrcs/rdgs/attach/ainsworth.1979.amer_psych.pdf. (Accessed: 10 June 2018).

Axline, V. M. (1989) *Play Therapy*. London: Churchill Livingstone.

Bamford, J. & Akhurst, J. (2014) 'She's Not Going to Leave Me' – Counsellor's Feelings on Ending Therapy With Children. *British Journal of Guidance and Counselling*, 42(5), pp. 458–471. London: Routledge.

Bowlby, J. (1969) *Attachment and Loss: Volume 1 Attachment. Tavistock Institute of Human Relations*. Basic Books. Available at: www.abebe.org.br/files/John-Bowlby-Attachment-Second-Edition-Attachment-and-Loss-Series-Vol-1-1983.pdf (Accessed: 10 June 2018).

Bowlby, J. (1988) *A Secure Base: Parent-Child Attachment and Healthy Human Development*. London: Routledge. Available at: file:///F:/dissertation%20proposal/How%20the%20Play%20Therapist%20manages%20the%20ending%20when%20considering%20attachment%20relationship/Evidence%20for%20attachment%20relationships%20in%20therapy/John-Bowlby-A-Secure-Base-Parent-Child-A.pdf. (Accessed: 10 June 2018).

Campbell, V. A., Baker, D. B. & Bratton, S. (2000) Why Do Children Drop Out From Play Therapy? *Clinical Child Psychology and Psychiatry*, 5(1), pp. 133–138. Available at: http://journals.sagepub.com/doi/abs/10.1177/1359104500005001013?journalCode=ccpa. (Accessed: 10 June 2018).

Cangelsoi, D. (1997) *Saying Goodbye in Child Psychotherapy: Planned, Unplanned & Premature Endings*. London: Jason Aronson Inc.

Clausen, J. M., Ruff, S. C., Wierderhold, W. V. & Heineman, T. V. (2012) For as Long as It Takes: Relationship Based Play Therapy for Children in Foster Care. *Psychoanalytic Social Work*, 19(1–2), pp. 43–53. Available at: www.tandfonline.com/doi/abs/10.1080/15228878.2012.666481. (Accessed: 10 June 2018).

Cochran, N. H., Nordling, W. & Cochran, J. L. (2010) *Child-Centred Play Therapy: A Practical Guide to Developing Therapeutic Relationships with Children*. New York: John Wiley & Sons.

Dighton, R. (2001) Towards a Definition of Play Therapy (Part 1). *Play Therapy: BAPT Newsletter*, 28, pp. 8–11. Surrey: British Association of Play Therapists.

Hughes, D. (2006) *Building the Bonds of Attachment: Awakening Love in Deeply Troubled Children* (3rd ed.). Washington: Rowman & Littlefield.

Landreth, G. L. (2002) *Play Therapy: The Art of the Relationship* (2nd ed.). Hove: Brunner-Routledge.

Lanyado, M. (2004) *The Presence of The Therapist: Treating Childhood Trauma*. East Sussex: Brunner-Routledge.

Mallinckrodt, B., Coble, H. M. & Gantt, D. M. (1995) Attachment Patterns in the Psychotherapy Relationship: Development of the Client Attachment to Therapist Scale. *Journal of Counselling Psychology. US: American Psychological Association*, 42(3), pp. 318–320. Available at: http://journals.sagepub.com/doi/abs/10.1177/0265407509360905. (Accessed: 10 June 2018).

Marmarosh, C. L. (2017) Fostering Engagement During Termination: Applying Attachment Theory and Research. *Psychotherapy: American Psychological Association. US: Educational Publishing Foundation*, 54(1), pp. 4–9.

Myrick, A. (2017) *Engaging Parents in Adolescent Therapy: Beyond the Waiting Room.* London: Rowman & Littlefield.

Norcross, J. C., Zimmerman, B. E., Greenberg, R. P. & Swift, J. K. (2017) Do All Therapists Do That When Saying Goodbye? A Study of Commonalities in Termination Behaviours. *Psychotherapy: American Psychological Association. US: Educational Publishing Foundation*, 54 (1), pp. 66–75.

Nordling, W. J. & Guerney, L. (1999) Typical Stages in the Child-Centred Play Therapy Process *The Journal for the Professional Counsellor*, 14(1), pp. 17–24.

Oaklander, V. (2007) *Windows to Our Children: A Gestalt Therapy Approach to Children and Adolescents.* Maine: The Gestalt Journal Press.

O'Connor, K. J. & Schaefer, C. E. (eds.) (1994) *Handbook of Play Therapy: Volume Two: Advances and Innovations.* New York: John Wiley & Sons, Inc.

Ray, D. C. (2014) Endings. In: Pattison, S., Robinson, M. & Beynon, A. (eds.) *The Handbook of Counselling Children and Young People* (pp. 229–244). London: Sage.

Sloves, R. E. & Bellinger Peterlin, K. (1994) Time Limited Play Therapy. In: O'Connor, K. & Schaefer, C. E. (eds.) *Handbook of Play Therapy. Volume Two: Advances and Innovations.* New York: John Wiley & Sons, Inc.

Smith, J. A. & Eatough, V. (2007) Interpretative Phenomenological Analysis. In: Lyons, E. & Coyle, A. (eds.) *Analysing Qualitative Data in Psychology* (pp. 35–50). London: Sage Publications Ltd.

West, J. (1996) *Child Centred Play Therapy* (2nd ed.). London: Arnold.

Wheeldon, M. (2018) *When We Say "Goodbye": An Investigation Into Play Therapists' Experiences of Endings Using Interpretative Phenomenological Analysis.* Surrey: Roehampton University Research Project.

# Index

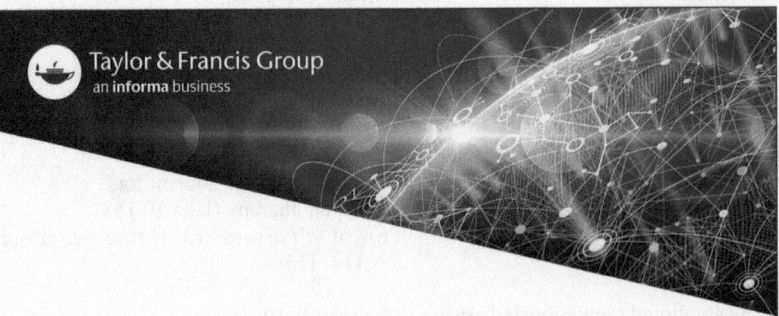
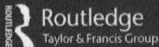
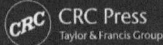